Other titles from Sweet Ch'i Press
of interest to readers of this book:

Master Cheng's Thirteen Chapters On T'ai-chi ch'üan
Cheng Man-ch'ing's Advanced T'ai-chi Form
  Instructions with Selections on Meditation,
  Medicine, the I ching and the Arts
The Healing Herbs of China (chart)

T'ai-chi Touchstones:

Yang Family Secret Transmissions

楊家太極拳秘訣

*Compiled and translated
by Douglas Wile*

Cover portraits, top to bottom:
Yang Chein-hou, Yang Shao-hou, Yang Ch'eng-fu

Published by
Sweet Ch'i Press
662 Union St.
Brooklyn, New York 11215

15 14 13

Acknowledgments

From each according to his abilities;
to each my heartfelt gratitude:

Louis Alfalla, William Brown, Janet Christie,
William Foley, Hung Ming-shui, Lee Ch'ing-tse,
Zack Rogow, John Salerno, P. David Weiss

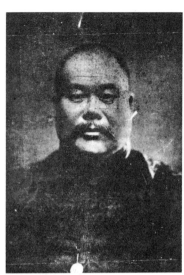

Yang Ch'eng-fu

Fourth Anniversary
Gathering of the
Chih Jou T'ai-chi ch'üan
Association, 1929.▶

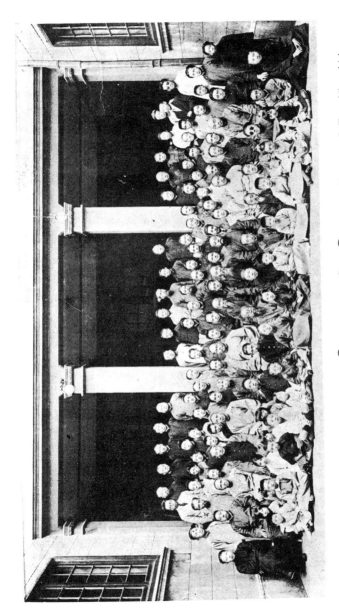

1. Yang Ch'eng-fu   3. Sun Lu-t'ang   5. Tung Ying-chieh
2. Yang Shao-hou   4. Wu Chien-ch'üan   6. Ch'en Wei-ming

Translator's Note

T'ai-chi ch'üan, although it defies categorization, may be succinctly defined as the spirit of Chinese metaphysics, meditation, and medicine in the body of a martial art. Theories regarding the origins of this soft-style or "internal" art have been essentially of two kinds: the mythic and the humanistic. The mythic, or *yang*, approach involves the giving of the art by an inspired sage or immortal, whereas the humanistic, or *yin*, approach emphasizes the painstaking process of cultural evolution. Even modern scholars may differ as widely as Ch'en Kung, who typifies the mythic mode,

> Whether Chang San-feng or someone else, whoever invented this subtle and profound martial art must have been an ancient Taoist possessed of the highest wisdom and could not possibly have been a common man. [1]

and T'ang Hao, who represents the humanistic attitude,

> Historical records and investigations in the field reveal that t'ai-chi ch'üan was created during the late Ming and early Ch'ing, or approximately 300 years ago. It combined and developed the various boxing styles that were popular among the people and the army during the Ming and added to this the ancient *tao-yin* and breathing techniques, absorbing classical materialist philosophy, *yin-yang* theory, and medical knowledge concerning circulation of the blood and *ch'i* to form a martial art, that trains both the external and internal. [2]

These two modes of conceptualization—legend and history—need not be mutually exclusive, but they should not be confused. Human experience is enriched by myth and legend just as surely as it is not impoverished by knowledge of mundane history. Nevertheless, considered in the context of the social and intellectual history of China during the first half of this century, these two approaches reflect a more fundamental split in political philosophies: the one based on idealism, elitism, and hero worship and the other based on materialism, egalitarianism, and the self-confidence of the masses.

The origins controversy rages unabated even today, though the battle lines are not so neatly drawn along the Taiwan Straits. With greater freedom of expression on both Taiwan and Mainland China, one now hears pro-Chang San-feng voices from the Mainland and supporters of the strictly historical approach from Taiwan. New claims to be the true cradle of t'ai-chi ch'üan have emerged from Hung-tung County in Shansi and Chao-pao Village in Honan, the former using mainly historical analysis and the latter constructing a lineage from Chang San-feng to Chiang Fa to Ch'en Ch'ing-p'ing. Students of the history of t'ai-chi ch'üan face a growing base of primary materials and an exploding range of secondary sources, even as we learn to read between the lines for the biases of lineage, ideology, and commercialism.

If we cannot be certain of the early phase of t'ai-chi's genesis and transmission, scholars generally agree that the goods must somehow be delivered to or developed by the Ch'en family of Ch'en Village (Ch'en-chia-kou), Honan, where they were picked up by Yang Fu-k'uei (Lu-ch'an, 1799-1872) in the early 19th century. Geographically, t'ai-chi ch'üan spread in a series of widening circles. From Ch'en Village it was transmitted to Yung-nien County in Hopeh, and then to Peking in the North, Nanking, Shanghai, Hangchow, Wuhan and Canton in the South, the other provinces of the littoral and hinterlands, Hongkong, overseas Chinatowns, and finally non-Chinese students. Centripedal forces limiting the diffusion of t'ai-chi ch'üan prior to the 20th century—feudalism, the family system, and a foreign dynasty—gave way to centrifugal forces calling for a revival of martial fitness to throw off Manchu rule and counter Japanese, Russian, and Western imperialism.

Who were these men who devoted themselves so unstintingly to the martial arts, and what were their motives. Some were simply bodyguards and bullies for the rich landlords, and some were men who fought for righteous causes. These causes might be as local as avenging victims of family feuds or as national as revolution and racial salvation. The story of t'ai-chi's rise in the late 19th and early 20th century has its plot and its characters. The plot is China's need for self-strengthening, and the cast of characters begins with Yang Lu-ch'an.

The Founder: Yang Lu-ch'an

There are two major versions of Yang Lu-ch'an's background — one "official" and the other probably historical. The "official" version emanates from colleagues and students who may have wished to conceal his humble origins. Hsü Yü-sheng, student of Lu-ch'an's son, Chien-hou (1839-1917), and author of *Illustrated Manual of T'ai-chi Ch'üan* (T'ai-chi ch'üan shih t'u-chieh) published in 1921, says that Lu-ch'an along with fellow Yung-nien villager, Li Po-k'uei, on hearing of Ch'en Ch'ang-hsing's fame as a martial artist, made haste to Ch'en Village to study with him. Initially regarded as outsiders, they won over the master by sheer determination and finally gained the complete transmission, whereupon they returned to Yung-nien. Lu-ch'an later traveled to Peking, where he became martial arts tutor to the Manchu nobility.[3] Ch'en Wei-ming, student of Lu-ch'an's grandson, Ch'eng-fu, in his 1925 *Art of Tai-chi Chüan* (T'ai-chi ch'üan shu) closely follows Hsü's account, adding a few embellishments. Ch'en tells us that after arriving in Ch'en Village, Yang heard loud sounds issuing from a nearby building. Climbing a wall, he poked a hole in a window and spied Ch'ang-hsing giving instruction in uprooting. By nightly surveillance he learned all the secrets, and when the master finally consented to accept him as a student, he made such rapid progress that he soon surpassed even the Ch'en family favorites.[4] Thus Yang Ch'eng-fu's preface to his 1934 *Complete Principles and Applications of T'ai-chi Ch'üan* (T'ai-chi ch'üan t'i-yung ch'üan-shu), probably ghost-written by Cheng Man-ch'ing,[5] contains biographical information about the Yang family, that not only respectfully glosses over Lu-ch'an's background, but puts in the illiterate 19th century Lu-ch'an's mouth the world view and political agenda of the early 20th century conservative intelligentsia, even fabricating an anachronistic dialogue between Ch'eng-fu and his grandfather, Lu-ch'an, who actually died eleven years before his grandson's birth. Ch'eng-fu's account here, or more likely that of his ghost-writer, has Lu-ch'an traveling to Ch'en Village as a adult on the strength of Ch'ang-hsing's reputation, and remaining for ten years before being accepted as a student.[6] Ch'en Kung's 1943 *T'ai-chi Hand Form, Broadsword, Two-Edged Sword, Spear and Sparring* (T'ai-chi ch'üan tao chien kan san-shou ho-pien) is a remake of Ch'en Wei-ming's account, except that he has Lu-ch'an going to Ch'en Village as a young boy and making a hole in the wall, that he claims could still be seen in the 1940's.[7]

Even the great martial arts scholar, Hsü Chen, fell under the spell of Yang family well-wishers in his 1930 *Summary of Chinese Martial Arts* (Kuo-chi lun-yüeh), uncritically reproducing Hsü Yü-sheng's account.[8] However, just six years later in his *A Study of the Truth of T'ai-chi Ch'üan* (T'ai-chi ch'üan k'ao-hsin lu) Hsü Chen finally breaks the taboo. It was Hsü whose teacher, Hao Yüeh-ju, first showed him Li I-yü's handwritten copies of Wu Yü-hsiang's manuscripts. Noting that Li's "Short Preface to T'ai-chi Ch'üan" (T'ai-chi ch'üan hsiao-hsü) referred to Yang Lu-ch'an as "a certain Yang of Nan-kuan," Hsü resolved to examine the reason for this circumlocution. After interviewing the older generation of martial arts enthusiasts in Yung-nien, Ch'en Village, and Peking, he discovered that the Ch'en family owned a pharmacy in Yung-nien, the Hall of Great Harmony (T'ai-ho t'ang). The proprietor of the pharmacy, Ch'en Te-hu, was one of the richest men in Ch'en Village and he hired one of his clansmen, Ch'en Ch'ang-hsing, to teach his sons the martial arts. After many years of waiting on Ch'ang-hsing, Lu-ch'an absorbed much of the art, and when he began to prompt Ch'ang-hsing's students, the master was so impressed that he not only transmitted the art to him but bought his freedom for fifty ounces of silver and returned him to Yung-nien. Back in Yung-nien, Lu-ch'an stayed in the Ch'en family Hall of Harmony Pharmacy, whose local landlord was Wu Yü-hsiang and his two brothers. The Wu brothers were a prominent gentry family in Yung-nien, and keenly interested in the martial arts. Breaking class barriers, Yü-hsiang studied with Lu-ch'an, which whetted his appetite to seek out Lu-ch'an's teacher, Ch'en Ch'ang-hsing. On his way to Ch'en Village, Yü-hsiang passed through nearby Chao-pao Village, where the local innkeeper, who coveted Yü-hsiang's room and board, told him that Ch'en Ch'ing-p'ing was superior to Ch'ang-hsing and persuaded him to stay in Chao-pao. Hsü concludes that Li I-yü in his "Short Preface" attempted to protect the reputation of the Wu family by not revealing the fact that his uncle, Yü-hsiang, was initiated into t'ai-chi by a man so poor he had been sold as a bond servant.[9]

Wu Yü-hsiang's grandson, Wu Lai-hsü, in his "Biography of My Grandfather, Wu Lien-ch'üan" (Hsien wang-fu Lien-ch'üan fu-chün hsing-lüeh) shows a similar delicacy in handling the connection between Yang Lu-ch'an and the Wu family. Lai-hsü's biography states that Yü-hsiang, on learning of Ch'en Ch'ang-hsing's art, desired to study but could not get away from the capital, and so sent Yang Lu-ch'an to Ch'en Village in his stead to investigate. Later, Lai-hsü tells us, Wu went personally to Honan and studied with Ch'en Ch'ing-p'ing.[10] Hao Yin-ju's version has Ch'ing-p'ing agreeing to teach Wu Yü-hsiang in exchange for help in a legal entanglement. Ch'ing-p'ing was so ill at the time, however, that he instructed Wu from his sick bed.[11]

In 1930 Lu-ch'an's grandson, Yang Ch'eng-fu, while serving as Dean of Instruction at the Chekiang Martial Arts Institute, received an inquiry from the Central Martial Arts Institute regarding the birth and death dates of his late grandfather. In his response, Ch'eng-fu disclosed that Lu-ch'an began studying with Ch'ang-hsing at the age of ten and did not return to Yung-nien until in his forties.[12] This directly contradicts the Li I-yü and Wu Lai-hsü versions, and even those put into Ch'eng-fu's mouth by Hsü Yü-sheng, Ch'en Wei-ming, Tung Ying-chieh and Cheng Man-ch'ing. Of course, Ch'eng-fu does not explain how or why a poor boy of ten would travel to another province and live with an unrelated family for thirty years. Sung Fu-t'ing and Sung Chih-chien, supporters of the "poor boy" thesis, nevertheless rearrange many of the other details. They have Lu-ch'an initially employed as a servant in the Wu household in Yung-nien from whence he is sent to work in a Wu family pharmacy in Huai-ch'ing, Honan. The Ch'en's of Ch'en-chia-kou also operated a pharmacy in Huai-ch'ing, and when they advertised for a servant, Lu-ch'an jumped ship, eventually ending up under the roof of Ch'en Ch'ang-hsing. By spying and surreptitous training he surpassed Ch'ang-hsing's students and was accepted for the highest initiation. After two years of intensive study he requested his wages and returned to Yung-nien, where Wu Yü-hsiang in turn studied with his former servant for two years. Wu now traveled to Honan, and after studying with Ch'en Ch'ing-p'ing, made such progress that Yang became jealous and returned to Ch'ang-hsing for advanced instruction. Ch'ang-hsing gave him the transmissions of Chang Sang-feng, Chiang Fa and Wang Tsung-yüeh, and Lu-ch'an, realizing the Taoist origins of the art, journeyed to the Wu-tang Mountains in search of a master. It was here that he studied Taoist yoga and the soft aspect of martial arts and invented push-hands. Returning to the world as a comsummate martial artist, he was introduced by Wu Yü-hsiang in Peking.[13]

In the winter and spring of 1930-31, China's pioneer and most prolific martial arts historian, T'ang Hao, traveled to Ch'en Village on a mission to solve this and many other mysteries in the history of t'ai-chi ch'üan. T'ang interviewed Ch'en Ch'eng-wu, the grandson of Ch'en Te-hu, owner of the pharmacy in Yung-nien and the one who bought Lu-ch'an as a servant. According to Ch'eng-wu, martial arts master Ch'en Ch'ang-hsing's house being rather small and rustic, he instructed his clansmen in the main hall of Te-hu's house. When Te-hu died, he left behind a widow, whose relatively young age made it unseemly for Lu-ch'an to continue to live in the house. As a result, Lu-ch'an's bond papers were burned and he was sent back to Yung-nien.[14] This tallies with Hsü Chen's findings, and both scholars explain the cover-up of Yang Lu-ch'an's origins as a relic of feudal class consciousness.

The most significant recent contribution to the Yang family record is that of centenarian, Wu T'u-nan, whose 1984 *Studies on T'ai-chi Ch'üan* (T'ai-chi ch'üan chih yen-chiu) describes his years of study with Wu Chien-ch'üan and Yang Shao-hou, his 1919 fieldwork in Ch'en-chia-kou, and interviews with principals in the martial arts renaissance during the early Republican period. Wu's version is unique in many respects and contradicts a number of points of relative agreement in other published accounts. Wu describes Yang

Lu-ch'an as a sick young man who traveled to Ch'en-chia-kou with money and provisions in search of a cure. Gaining both health and mastery of t'ai-chi ch'üan from Ch'en Ch'ang-hsing, he returned to Yung-nien where Wu Yü-hsiang approached him for instruction. Because of Wu's arrogance, Lu-ch'an sent his second son, Pan-hou, to instruct him. Wu was frustrated by his lack of progress and determined to appeal to Ch'en Ch'ang-hsing himself. Because of Ch'ang-hsing's advanced age, Wu studied with Ch'en Ch'ing-p'ing, returning to Yung-nien after little more than a month claiming to have grasped the secrets. Later Yü-hsiang made an enemy of a Shaolin monk, and hoping to get revenge, encouraged Lu-ch'an to challenge the monk to a match. When the monk died as a result of injuries sustained at Lu-ch'an's hands, the incident was reported to local officials, and Lu-ch'an was advised by Wu to lay low in the capital. Yü-hsiang's older brother, Ju-ch'ing (Cho-t'ang), served in the Ministry of Justice, and a friend in the Ministry, Chang Feng-ch'i, hosted the Yangs in his home. Chang also operated a large pickled vegetable factory, that was provisioner to the imperial household and a frequent stopover for Manchu princes returning from hunting expeditions. Lu-ch'an and sons ended up rotating between the households of Chang Feng-ch'i, Prince Tai-i, Prince Tai-chih, and the Manchu military academy so that none were ever without the tutorial services of a Yang Master. Wu T'u-nan reports that Tai-chih was the best of Lu-ch'an's students, and it was from discussions with Tai-chih and his son, P'u-t'ung, that Wu gleaned most of his information.[15]

An historical novel based on the life of Yang Lu-ch'an and published in occupied Tientsin in the early forties under the pen-name Pai Yü offers an interesting counterpoint to the accounts of students and scholars. The fictionalized Lu-ch'an, sickly son of a rich peasant, journeys to Honan as a young man in search of t'ai-chi master Ch'en Ch'ing-p'ing (not Ch'en Ch'ang-hsing). Repeatedly turned away by the master, he resorts to disguising himself as a mute mendicant and after years of sweeping Ch'ing-p'ing's doorstep finally melts the master's heart and is accepted as a student. Completing his training with Ch'ing-p'ing, he goes to Peking, where after fighting pa-kua founder, Tung Hai-ch'uan, to a stand-off, he challenges the whole capital martial arts establishment. After defeating all comers, he reigns supreme until his death, when son and heir apparent, Pan-hou, is bested by his father's student, Wang Lan-t'ing. Pan-hou, disgraced, trains for ten years to restore the honor of the family name. Later Pan-hou became an opium addict, but despite his lack of strength was able to overcome the strongest opponents. When asked why the Kuang-p'ing students of the Yang family showed both hard and soft techniques in their style, whereas the Peking students showed only soft techniques, Pan-hou replied that the Peking students were mainly wealthy aristocrats, and that, after all, there was a difference between Chinese and Manchus, implying a policy of passive resistance to the alien dynasty by imparting only half the t'ai-chi ch'üan transmission.[16]

Readers may draw their own conclusions from these widely divergent accounts of Lu-ch'an's background. T'ang Hao tells us that he himself the son of a poor peasant and a man who rose from poverty to become a famous lawyer and pre-eminent martial arts historian was the object of a nearly successful conspiracy to silence him for his efforts to demythologize the orgins of t'ai-chi ch'üan. Examining motives, it is easy in the context of a highly stratified feudal society to understand the sensibilities of Yang family members and their partisans. By the same logic, were Ch'en and Hao informants attempting to diminish Yang's reputation by exposing his origins? This is less clear. Historians, Hsü and T'ang, were bent on setting the record straight, both out of scholarly scrupples and to strike a blow at feudal class consciousness. If Hsü and T'ang's research is correct, however, no fictional account of Lu-ch'an's background could be as stirring as the story of a slave boy who became martial arts master to the Manchu princes, foremost boxer throughout the empire, and founder of a lineage that dominates a worldwide movement.

The Transmission: Four Generations of Yangs

Of the many hand forms listed in the Ch'en family manuals, by the time of Ch'en Ch'ang-hsing in the late 18th and early 19th century, only the first and second forms were still practiced. Ch'ang-hsing's style is further designated as "old" (*lao*) and "large" (*ta*), to distinguish it from the innovative "new" (*hsin*) and "small" (*hsiao*) style developed by Ch'ang-hsing's contemporary Ch'en Yu-pen and younger clansmen, Ch'en Ch'ing-p'ing. As a student of Ch'ang-hsing, what Lu-ch'an learned and presumably taught was the "old" and "large " versions of the First Form (Thirteen Postures) and Second Form (*p'ao-ch'ui*). According to Hsü Yü-sheng, the people of Yung-nien referred to Lu-ch'an's art as "Soft Boxing" (*juan-ch'üan*) or "Transformation Boxing" (*hua-ch'üan*).[17] Stylistically, the first two generations of Yangs retained much of the flavor of the Ch'en style. This judging from Ch'en Wei-ming's account of Yang Shao-hou's report of his father Lu-ch'an's ability to pluck a coin from the ground with his mouth during Single Whip Lower Style and to shoulder-stroke an opponent's knee and from Pan-hou's withering shouts while issuing energy.[18] This also explains the somewhat "harder" tone of Pan-hou's transmissions featured in Chapter V of the present anthology. Although it was the "old" and "large" Ch'en

Style that Lu-ch'an introduced to Wu Yü-hsiang on his return to Yung-nien, Wu subsequently studied the "new, small" style with Ch'en Ch'ing-p'ing and developed his own "small" style, as indicated by the accounts of students of Hao Yüeh-ju.

In his *Self-Defense Applications of T'ai-chi Ch'üan* (T'ai-chi ch'üan shih-yung fa), Yang Ch'eng-fu tells us that his grandfather, Lu-ch'an, was introduced in Peking by Wu Ju-ch'ing, Wu Yü-hsiang's older brother and a third degree (*chin-shih*) holder in the imperial examinations of 1840. Wang Hsin-wu, a student of Wu Chien-ch'üan and Hsü Yü-sheng, in his 1942 *Exposition of T'ai-chi Ch'üan* (T'ai-chi ch'üan fa ch'an-tsung) describes mid 19th century Peking and the Manchu custom of patronizing men of unusual talent. Lu-ch'an as the foremost martial artist in Peking was retained by no fewer then eight Manchu princes, and so was nicknamed not only "Yang the Invincible," but also "Eight Lords."[19]

Lu-ch'an's sons, Yü (Pan-hou, 1837-1892) and Chien (Chien-hou, 1839-1917), were worthy successors. So rigorous was the training regimen under their father that it is reported Pan-hou tried to run away from home and Chien-hou attempted suicide.[20] In spite of their shared childhood experiences, they developed opposite natures. Pan-hou was said to be brutal in demonstrating his prowess, sparing not even his own students. His only son, Chao-p'eng, chose to pursue farming in Yung-nien. Chien-hou by contrast, was gentle and affable and attracted many students. Wang Hsin-wu tells us that Lu-ch'an, Pan-hou and Chien-hou often stayed in the residence of Prince Tuan, where they taught t'ai-chi ch'üan. Rival soft-stylists, Tung Hai-ch'uan boarded with Prince Su, where he taught pa-kua, and Kuo Yung-ch'en with Duke Yü, where he taught hsing-i. Later, Li Shih-chün served as martial arts trainer at the Eastern Garrison in Peking, while Pan-hou served in the Western Garrison. Rivalry between the two garrisons at this time did much to spur the resurgence of China's martial arts and the martial spirit in general.[21] Pan-hou was also influenced by family friend Wu Yü-hsiang and his form has been classified as "small " style, whereas his brother, Chien-hou, reached a compromise and his style is called "middle" (*chung*). Lu-ch'an and Pan-hou's best student was the Manchu, Ch'üan Yu (1834-1902), whose son Wu Chien-ch'üan (1870-1942) was the founder of the Wu style. Hsü Yü-sheng, a student of Chien-hou, reports that of Lu-ch'an's students in the Manchu garrisons the best were Wan Ch'un, Ling Shan, and Ch'üan Yu, each of whom developed one aspect of Lu-ch'an's skill—hardness, repelling, and neutralizing—but only Lu-ch'an himself possessed all three in equal measure and superiority.[22]

Chien-hou sired two successors, Chao-hsiung (Meng-hsiang, Shao-hou, 1862-1930) and Chao-ch'ing (Ch'eng-fu, 1883-1936), who both reverted to the expansive "large" style, although Shao-hou taught the compact "small" style as well. Ch'eng-fu's student, Huang Wen-shu, describing the styles of the two brothers, calls Shao-hou's style, "small and hard...fast and rooted," and Ch'eng-fu's, "open and soft...a bullet within cotton."[23] Not until late in Ch'eng-fu's career did retentions of the Ch'en style jumps, flying kicks, stamps, changes of pace, and shouts finally disappear from his form. In a 1990 interview shortly before his death, martial artist and martial arts historian Ku liu-hsin, recalled his impressions of Ch'eng-fu and Shao-hou. Ch'eng-fu, though an imposing figure of 300 pounds in his later years, was good-natured and popular with students, whereas Shao-hou,like his uncle Pan-hou, refused to pull punches even with rich and famous students and thus had a very small following.[24] So great was Ch'eng-fu's prestige, Huang Han-hsüan tells us, that the governor of Canton offered him 800 silver dollars a month to come south, and even generals humbled themselves before him.[25]

Wu T'u-nan, who in 1984 called himself the only living disciple of Yang Shao-hou, describes Lu-ch'an as large and powerfully built, Pan-hou as tall, thin and handsome, and Chien-hou somewhere in-between. Wu makes reference to a secret Yang form for advanced applications comprising more than two hundred movements performed in only three minutes.[26] Of Ch'eng-fu's four sons, perhaps Chen-ming (Shou-chung) and Chen-to did most to pass on their father's art, though never exerting the international influence of Ch'eng-fu's intellectual disciples, Tung Ying-chieh and Cheng Man-ch'ing.

If the Ch'en style spawned the Yang style, all subsequent styles owe their origins directly or indirectly to Yang influence. The Wu style of Wu Chien-ch'üan came through Ch'üan Yu, a student of Yang Pan-hou. Although there is no record of how long Wu Yü-hsiang studied with Yang Lu-ch'an, his grandson tells us that he spent only a little more than a month with Ch'en Ch'ing-p'ing. Certainly it was Lu-ch'an who first introduced Wu to the art. Wu transmitted the art to Li I-yü, and Li to Hao Ho (Wei-chen, 1849-1920). Wu's style is in fact better known as the Hao style, after Hao Wei-chen and his son, Yüeh-ju (1877-1935). Hao Ho's student, Sun Lu-t'ang (1862-1932), in turn became the founder of the Sun style.

In 1956 the Martial Arts Division of the National Physical Education Committee of the People's Republic, in an effort to cut through stylistic rivalries and facilitate popularization, published their *Simplified T'ai-chi Ch'üan* (Chien-hua t'ai-chi ch'üan) introducing a twenty-four posture form based on twenty of Yang Ch'eng-fu's thirty-four distinct postures. This was followed in 1957 by their *Tai-chi Ch'üan Exercise* (T'ai-chi ch'üan yün-tung), which created a standard long form of eighty-eight postures, also based on Yang Ch'eng-fu's model. These developments institutionalized the Yang style and assured its dominance through the 1970's, after which there was a resurgence of family lineages and stylistic diversity.

It was through the Ch'en and Wu families that Yang Lu-ch'an was catapulted from humble status to darling of the Manchu princes; it was through Ch'eng-fu's educated disciples that t'ai-chi was adapted for practice by intellectuals, the sick, the elderly, and women. The Yang family thus became the vehicle by which conservative intellectuals could reconcile both the need for self-strengthening and the preservation of traditional culture and progressive intellectuals could embrace a wholesome legacy from the feudal past. In the words of martial arts poet, Yang Chi-tzu (1886-1965),

> Who would have thought that the
> art of the Ch'en's of Honan
> Would be given to the world
> by the Yang's of Hopeh.[27]

The Literary Tradition: Yang Family Classics

Just as the Yangs were not the creators but the transmitters and adaptors of t'ai-chi ch'üan, similarly their role in the transmission of the classics was not as authors but disseminators and commentators. Of the fourteen early 20th century editions of the Yang family transmission of the classics surveyed by Hsü Chen, he judges those of Kung Jun-t'ien, Ch'en Wei-ming, Wu Chien-ch'üan, and Li Hsien-wu to be the least tampered with.[28] The core classics in these editions (by their Yang transmission titles) are the "T'ai-chi Ch'üan Classic," "Wang Tsung-yüeh's Treatise on T'ai-chi Ch'üan," "The Song of the Thirteen Postures," "The Mental Elucidation of the Practice of T'ai-chi Ch'üan," and "The Song of Sparring." Yang Lu-ch'an's illiteracy, together with the absence of all but the last of these texts in Ch'en Village, leaves only one source for these classics—Wu Yü-hsiang. Li I-yü's "Postscript to the T'ai-chi Ch'üan Classics" (T'ai-chi ch'üan pa) tells us that Wu himself found these texts in a salt shop in Wu-yang County, Honan.[29] The role of Chang San-feng in the composition of these works has been intensively studied and dismissed by most scholars since T'ang Hao's groundbreaking *Study of Shaolin and Wutang* (Shao-lin Wu-tang k'ao), published in 1930. More recently, even the historicity of Wang Tsung-yüeh has been questioned as more attention is focused on Wu Yü-hsiang's role in writing the classics and that of his nephew, Li I-yü, in compiling, editing, and augmenting them.[30]

If Wu Yü-hsiang himself composed the classics, as has been suggested, under the theoretical influence of Sung Dynasty metaphysician, Chou Tun-i, and Ch'ing martial arts commentator, Ch'ang Nai-chou, and under the practical influence of Lu-ch'an and Ch'en Ch'ing-p'ing, then these texts came into being during Lu-ch'an's lifetime and do not predate him.[31] If on the other hand, we accept the authenticity of the *Yin-fu Spear and T'ai-chi Ch'üan Manuals*, that T'ang Hao found in the Peking bookstalls as genuinely that of Wang Tsung-yüeh,[32] and also accept the authenticity of Li I-yü's "Postscript," that identifies the source of the Wu family manuscripts as the salt shop in Wu-yang,[33] then the discussion must turn to an exploration of the relationship between Wang Tsung-yüeh and the Ch'en family of Ch'en Village. On this point, the two greatest scholars of the history of Chinese martial arts—Hsü Chen and T'ang Hao—hold diametric views, Hsü believing that Wang Tsung-yüeh brought the art to Ch'en Village, and T'ang Hao that he received it there.[34] Questions regarding the authorship and authenticity of these texts do not alter the fact that Yang Lu-ch'an could only have received them from Wu Yü-hsiang.

If Yang Lu-ch'an received the classics from student

and patron, Wu Yü-hsiang, how do we account for differences between the Wu and Yang versions? Hsü Chen attributes these differences to the Yang version representing an earlier redaction of the Wu manuscripts than the Li I-yü copies.[35] Hsü further explains the crediting of Chang San-feng as the creator of t'ai-chi ch'üan in Yang sources to overzealous student's attempts to hyperbolize the art by giving it fabulous origins. T'ang Hao, however, rejects this interpretation, pointing out that the earliest of the extant Li I-yü manuscripts, the 1867 copy of Ma T'ung-wen, as well as the biographies of Wu Yü-hsiang by his grandsons, Wu Lai-hsü and Wu Yen-hsü, all attribute the art to the Immortal Chang. Thus according to T'ang, Yang was simply parroting the story he heard from Wu's own lips.[36]

The earliest published form manuals based on the Yang transmission were not of Yang authorship. Hsü Yü-sheng, student of Chien-hou and founder during the late Ch'ing of the Peking Physical Education Research Institute, published what must be considered the first modern manual on t'ai-chi ch'üan in 1921, the *Illustrated Manual of T'ai-chi Ch'üan*. Ch'eng-fu's student, Ch'en Wei-ming, followed this in 1925 with his *Art of T'ai-chi Ch'üan*, featuring photographs of Ch'eng-fu, Ch'en Wei-ming himself, and even Hsü Yü-sheng demonstrating Push-hands with Ch'eng-fu. Finally in 1931, *Self-Defense Methods of T'ai-chi Ch'üan* was published in Ch'eng-fu's own name. Yang's educated students were embarrassed by its lack of literary polish, and it was quickly withdrawn from circulation. A more complete and definitive edition of Ch'eng-fu's teachings was compiled and published under the title *Complete Principles and Applications of T'ai-chi Ch'üan* in 1934. Cheng Man-ch'ing's 1946 *Master Cheng's Thirteen Chapters on T'ai-chi Ch'üan* (Cheng-tzu t'ai-chi ch'üan shih-san p'icn) paid homage to his teacher, Yang Ch'eng-fu, even while modifying the form and elaborating the theory. Each of these works is represented in the present collection. Chapter VI of this anthology features fourteen texts copied from a manuscript containing a total of forty-three, that Shen Chia-chen copied from Yang Ch'eng-fu, and Ku Liu-hsin published in his *Studies on T'ai-chi Ch'üan* (T'ai-chi ch'üan yen-chiu) in 1963. Although the disposition of the remaining twenty-nine texts is unknown to the present writer, this may be one direction from which to look for future releases.

To date, then, this collection encompasses the totality of reprinted material handed down by three generations of Yang family masters. The first three chapters of this collection represent the latest stage in the Yang family transmission, transcriptions by students of Yang Ch'eng-fu's oral instructions. Their familiar narrative form makes them readily accessible to Western readers, and for this reason they have been introduced at the beginning. Chapters IV through VI contain material in the "secret transmissions" (*chüeh*) form. These consist of short aphoristic formulae and mnemonic verses composed as training songs to facilitate memorization and encode the essence of movement and applications. The final chapters, VII and VIII, are a collection of biographical literature, notes on the classics, and miscellaneous comments. Though gathered from many sources, taken together these fragments add up to whole cloth and have a consistency of both principle and spirit. As a unified thrust spanning a century of development, they clearly belong together.

Prof. Douglas Wile
Brooklyn College
Spring, 1993

Notes

1. Ch'en Kung. 1943. *T'ai-chi ch'üan tao chien kan san-shou ho-pien* (T'ai-chi hand form, broadsword, two-edged sword, spear and sparring). Hongkong: Chien-shen ch'u-pan-she (reprint, n.d.), p. 10.

2. T'ang Hao, Ku Liu-hsin. 1963. *T'ai-chi ch'üan yen-chiu* (A study of t'ai-chi ch'üan). Hongkong: Pai-ling ch'u-pan-she, p. 5.

3. Hsü Yü-sheng. 1921. T'ai-chi ch'üan shih t'u-chieh (Illustrated manual of t'ai-chi ch'üan). Hongkong: Hsiang-kang chin-hua ch'u-pan-she (reprint, n.d.), pp. 7-10. Also excerpted in Li T'ien-chi, ed., 1988. *Wu-tang chüeh-chi* (The martial arts of Wutang). Kirin: Chi-lin k'o-hsüeh ch'u-pan-she, pp. 273-75.

4. Ch'en Wei-ming. 1925. *Tai-chi ch'üan shu* (The art of t'ai-chi ch'üan). Hongkong: Hsiang-kang wu-shu ch'u-pan-she (reprint, n.d.), pp. 3-4.

5. See Chang Tun-hsi. 1975. "T'ai-chi ch'üan fa-chan yü chu-shu" (The development of t'ai-chi ch'üan and bibliography of writings). *Chung-kuo wu-shu shih-liao chi-k'an*, Vol. 2, p. 48; Li Min-ti. "T'an Yang-shih t'ai-chi ch'üan te chi-ke tung-tso ming-ch'eng" (A discussion of some of the names for postures in Yang style t'ai-chi ch'üan). *Wu-lin* 87 (1988), p. 16.

6. Yang Ch'eng-fu. 1934. *Tai-chi ch'üan t'i-yung ch'üan-shu* (Complete principles and applications of t'ai-chi ch'üan). Taipei: Chung-hua wu-shu ch'u-pan-she (reprint, 1975), pp. 3-4.

7. Ch'en Kung, *T'ai-chi ch'üan tao chien kan san-shou ho-pien*, p. 11.

8. Hsü chen. 1930. *Kuo-chi lun-lüeh* (Summary of Chinese martial arts). Shanghai: Commercial Press, pp. 53-54.

9. Hsü Chen. 1936. *T'ai-chi ch'üan k'ao-hsin lu* (A study of the truth of t'ai-chi ch'üan). In Teng Shih-hai, ed. 1980 *Tai-chi ch'üan kao* (Studies on t'ai-chi ch'üan). Hongkong: Tung-ya t'u-shu kung-ssu, pp. 120-21.

10. Li Fu-k'uei, ed., *Lien-jang t'ang pen tai-chi ch'üan p'u*. In *Tai-chi ch'üan yen-chiu*, pp. 152-53.

11. Hao Yin-ju. 1992. "T'ai-chi che-jen—chi-nien Wu Yü-hsiang tan-ch'en 180 chou-nien" (The philospher of t'ai-chi ch'üan—in commemoration of the 180th anniversarv of Wu Yü-hsiang's birthday). *Chung-hua wu-shu* 8 (1992),p. 30.

12. T'ang Hao. *T'ai-chi ch'üan yen-chiu*, p. 154. See also T'ang Hao. 1986. *Shen-chou wu-i* (Martial arts of China). Ch'ang-ch'un, Kirin: Chi-lin wen-shih ch'u-pan-she, p. 184.

13. Sung Fu-t'ing, Sung Chih-chien. 1966. "T'ai-chi ch'üan Yang tsu-shih Lu-ch'an chuan" (Biography of Yang Lu-ch'an). In *Tai-chi ch'üan yen-chiu chuan-chi* 22, pp. 19-21.

14. T'ang Hao. *T'ai-chi ch'üan yen-chiu*, p. 154.

15. Wu T'u-nan. 1984. *T'ai-chi ch'üan chih yen-chiu* (Studies on tai-chi ch'üan). Hongkong: Commercial Press, pp. 38-42.

16. Pai Yü. n.d. *Yang Lu-ch'an pieh-chuan* (The unofficial biography of Yang Lu-ch'an). Tienstin: Ch'ün-chi shu-chü.

17. Hsü Yü-sheng. *T'ai-chi ch'üan shih t'u-chieh*, p. 8.

18. Ch'en Wei-ming. 1929. *Tai-chi ch'üan ta-wen* (Questions and answers on t'ai-chi ch'üan). Taipei: T'ai-chi ch'üan hsüeh-shu yen-chiu hui, p. 14.

19. Quoted in Chang Tun-hsi. 1976. "T'ai-chi ch'üan yüan-liu tsai t'an-t'ao" (A further examination of the origins of t'ai-chi ch'üan). In *Chung-kuo wu-shu shih-liao chi-k'an*, Vol.3, pp. 48-52.

20. Ch'en Kung. *T'ai-chi ch'üan tao chien kan san-shou ho-pien*, p. 13.

21. Quoted in Chang Tun-hsi. 1976. "T'ai-chi ch'üan yüan-liu tsai t'an-t'ao" (A further examination of the origins of t'ai-chi ch'üan). In Chung-kuo wu-shu shih-liao chi-k'an, Vol. 3, p. 51.

22. Hsü Yü-sheng. *T'ai-chi ch'üan shih t'u-chieh*, p. 10 .

23. Huang Wen-shu, *Yang-chia t'ai-chi ch'üan ko-i yao-i*. Quoted in Chou Chien-nan. 1976. "T'ai-chi ch'üan li-shih te yen-chiu" (A study of the history of t'ai-chi ch'üan). In *Chung-kuo wu-shu shih-liao chi-k'an*, Vol.3, p. 89.

24. Yen Han-hsiu. 1991. "T'ai-chi ming-chia Ku Liu-hsin sheng-ch'ien i-hsi t'an" (A discussion with t'ai-chi master Ku Liu-hsin shortly before his death). *Wu-lin* 113, p. 24.

25. Huang Han-hsün. 1954. *Wu-lin chih-wen lu* (Anecdotes from the world of martial arts). Hongkong: T'ang-lang kuo-shu-kuan, p. 25.

26. Wu T'u-nan, *T'ai-chi ch'üan chih yen-chiu*, p. 100 .

27. Quoted in Ku Liu-hsin. 1982. *T'ai-chi ch'üan shu*. Shanghai: Shang-hai chiao-yü ch'u-pan-she, p. 362.

28. Hsü Chen. *T'ai-chi ch'üan k'ao-hsin lu*, pp. 98-105.

29. Ibid., pp. 174-75.

30. See Chao Hsi-min. 1976. *T'ai-chi ch'üan shih-san shih chih yen-chiu*. In *Chung-kuo wu-shu shih-liao chi-k'an*, Vol. 3, pp. 85-106; T.Y. Pang. 1987. *On Tai Chi Chuan*. Bellingham, Washington: Azalea Press, pp. 183.

31. Ibid.

32. T'ang Hao. 1935. *Wang Tsung-yüeh t'ai-chi ch'üan ching yen-chiu* (A study of Wang Tsung-yüeh's t'ai-chi ch'üan classics). Hongkong: Unicorn Press, p. 28.

33. Hsü Chen. *Tai-chi ch'üan kao-hsin lu*, pp. 78-90.

34. T'ang Hao. *Tai-chi ch'üan yen-chiu*, pp. 163-65.

35. Hsü Chen. *T'ai-chi ch'üan k'ao-hsin lu*, pp. 90-105.

36. T'ang Hao. *T'ai-chi ch'üan yen-chiu*, p. 163.

Table of Contents

Chapter I

A Discussion Of the Practice of T'ai-chi Ch'üan

Dictated by Yang Ch'eng-fu,
recorded by Chang Hung-k'uei
in Fu Chung-wen,
Yang-shih T'ai-chi ch'üan
(Yang style T'ai-chi ch'üan),
Hong Kong: T'ai-p'ing
shu-chü, 1971;
also Yang Ch'eng-fu,
*Yang-chia T'ai-chi ch'üan
t'i-yung ch'üan-shu*
(Yang family complete
principles and applications of
T'ai-chi ch'üan), Hong Kong:
Hsin-wen shu-tien, n.d.

Although there are innumerable schools within the Chinese martial arts, they are all based on philosophical principles. The ancients devoted whole lifetimes to them without being able to exhaust their marvels. Nevertheless, if students expend one day's effort, they will reap the benefits of one day. After many days and months one will naturally reach the goal. This art is not like track and field events in the West which are easily explained and demonstrated and require no subtle or profound study.

T'ai-chi ch'üan is the art of concealing hardness within softness, like a needle in cotton. Its technique, physiology and mechanics all involve considerable philosophical principles. Therefore students of this art must pass through definite stages of development over a long period of time. Although the guidance of a superior teacher and practice with fellow students is indispensable, the most important thing is one's own daily practice. One can discuss or dream a great deal, but when one day we are called upon to test our art, we will have nothing to show, for without daily discipline we will remain outsiders. This is why the ancients said, "Thought alone is without profit; it is much better to study." If one practices faithfully morning and evening, winter and summer, keeping the form always fresh, then regardless of age or sex, success is assured.

In recent years students of T'ai-chi ch'üan have traveled from the north of China to the south, from the Yellow River Valley to the Yangtze River Valley, and from the Yangtze to the Pearl River in Kwangtung. This increase in the number of enthusiasts is cause for great optimism for the future of our national martial arts. In coming years there will be no limit to the number of sincere and dedicated students. Although there is no shortage of students the majority fall into one of two erroneous paths. The first group are highly gifted, robust, quick witted and exceptionally penetrating, but unfortunately they are satisfied with small successes. Rapidly mastering the superficial, they abandon their studies and cannot learn a great deal. The second group consists of those who are eager for immediate results and careless of detail. Before a year is out they have already finished their study of the hand, two-edged sword, broadsword and spear forms. Although they are able to imitate the outer aspects of the form, in reality they are ignorant of its inner aspects. When we examine their direction and movements, the up and down, in and out, we find that they all fall short of the proper measure. If we try to make corrections, we find that every single posture requires correcting, and moreover the corrections made in the morning are already forgotten by evening. Therefore it is often said, ''The martial arts are easy to learn but difficult to correct.'' The origin of this saying lies in the desire for immediate results. Nowadays, errors are passed on as teachings and this must inevitably lead to self-delusion and deluding others. This is a cause of great concern for the future of the art.

At the very beginning of T'ai-chi ch'üan study, one first practices the form. What is meant by form study is careful memorization and imitation, under a teacher's guidance, of the individual posture in the form. Students must concentrate to calm their *ch'i* and quietly memorize, ponder and imitate the postures. This is called practicing the form. At this point students must pay special attention to distinguishing between internal and external, rising and descending. That which belongs to the internal is ''using the mind and not force.'' Descending means ''sinking the *ch'i* to the *tan-t'ien''* and rising refers to the ''light and sensitive energy at the top of the head.'' That which belongs to the external is the ''lightness and sensitivity of the whole body,'' ''the open connection of all the joints,'' ''from the feet to the legs to the waist,'' ''sinking the shoulders and folding

4

the elbows," and so forth. At the outset of study these teachings should be practiced morning and evening and thoroughly understood. Every posture and movement should be carefully analyzed. During actual practice, dedicate yourself to achieving correctness. When you master one posture, then go on to the next. In this way you will gradually acquire the whole form. If corrections are made step by step, then even after a long time there will be no change in the basic principles.

When practicing the movements, all the joints in the body should be relaxed and natural. First, one must not hold the breath. Second, the four limbs, the waist and legs must not use any strength. These two principles are recited by all martial artists of the internal systems. However, as soon as they begin to move, turning the body, kicking or rotating the waist, then they become out of breath and their bodies tremble. The cause is invariably holding the breath and using strength.

1. During practice the head must not incline to the side nor tilt up or down. This is what is meant by holding the head as if suspended from above, or the idea of balancing an object on top of the head. In order to avoid a stiff vertical posture, we emphasize the concept of suspension from above. Although the vision is straight ahead, it sometimes follows the movements of the body. Even though the line of vision is unfocused, it is nevertheless an important movement within the pattern of changes, and supplements deficiencies in body and hand techniques. The mouth seems open but is not open; it seems closed but it is not closed. Exhale through the mouth and inhale through the nose in a natural way. If saliva flows from beneath the tongue, it should occasionally be swallowed and not expelled.

2. The body should maintain an erect posture without leaning; spine and tailbone should hang in vertical alignment without inclining. Beginners must pay

special attention to this as they execute active movements involving opening and closing, relaxing the chest and raising the back, sinking the shoulders and turning the waist. Otherwise it will be difficult to correct this after a while and will lead to stiffness. Even though one may have devoted a great deal of time, there will be little benefit or practical advantage.

3. All the joints of the arms should be completely relaxed, with shoulders sunk and elbows folded down. The palms should be slightly extended and the fingertips slightly bent. Use the mind to move the arms and allow *ch'i* to reach the fingers. After many days and months the internal energy will become extremely sensitive and marvels will naturally manifest.

4. One must distinguish full and empty in the two legs. In rising and sinking one should move like a cat. If the weight of the body is shifted to the left leg, then the left leg is full and the right leg is empty. If the weight is shifted to the right leg, then the right leg is full and the left empty. What we mean by ''empty'' is not a vacuum, for there is no break in the potential for power, and the idea of extension and contraction remains. What we mean by ''full'' is simply that it is substantial and not that excessive force is used, for this would be considered brute strength. Therefore, when bending the legs, the foreleg should not extend beyond the vertical. To exceed this is considered an excess of energy. If when pushing forward we lose our vertical posture, our opponent will take advantage of this to attack us.

5. In regard to the feet, one must distinguish between kicking with the front of the foot (as in Separate Feet Left and Right or Spread Feet Left and Right in the form) and kicking with the heel. When kicking with the front of the foot, we must pay attention to the toes; when kicking with the heel pay attention to the sole of the foot.

Wherever the mind goes the *ch'i* will follow and wherever the *ch'i* goes there will naturally be energy. However, the joints of the leg should be completely relaxed and the kick should issue with evenness and stability. At this moment it is very easy to be guilty of using stiff force, wherein the body will rock and lack stability and the kick will have no power.

The T'ai-chi ch'üan curriculum consists of hand forms first (i.e., empty hand), such as T'ai-chi ch'üan and T'ai-chi Long Boxing. Next comes One Hand Push-Hands, Fixed Position Push-Hands, Push-Hands With Active Steps, Ta Lü, and Free Sparring. Last comes weapons, such as T'ai-chi Double-Edged Sword, T'ai-chi Broadsword, T'ai-chi Spear (Thirteen Spear), and so forth.

As for the length of practice, one should do two forms after rising in the morning, then do two more just before going to bed. Each day one should practice seven or eight times, and at the very least, once in the morning and once at night. However, avoid practice when drunk or after a meal.

As for the place of practice, courtyards or empty halls where there is sufficient air and light are best. Avoid strong winds or places which are dark, damp and foul smelling. This is because when we begin to move, the breathing becomes deeper, and if strong winds or foul air enter the body, it is injurious to the lungs and can easily lead to illness. As for clothing, loose fitting garments and wide-toed cloth shoes are best. If after practice one is sweating, avoid removing the clothes and standing naked or washing with cold water. Otherwise sickness is inevitable.

Chapter II

The Ten Important Points for T'ai-chi Ch'üan

Oral instructions of Yang Ch'eng-fu, recorded by Ch'en Wei-ming in *T'ai-chi ch'üan shu* (The art of T'ai-chi ch'üan), first published in 1925 by Ch'en's school, the Chih-jou ch'üan-she, reprinted by Hsiang-kang wu-shu ch'u-pan-she, Hong Kong, n.d.; also Yang Ch'eng-fu, *Yang-chia T'ai-chi ch'üan t'i-yung ch'üan-shu* (Yang family complete principles and applications of T'ai-chi ch'üan), Hong Kong: Hsin-wen shu-tien, n.d.

1. The Energy at the Top of the Head Should Be Light and Sensitive. "Energy at the top of the head" means that the head should be carried erect so that the spirit (*shen*) will reach to the very top. No strength should be used. If strength is used then the back of the neck will be stiff and the blood and *ch'i* will not be able to circulate. There should be a feeling of light sensitivity and naturalness. Without this light and sensitive energy at the top of the head, the spirit cannot rise up.

2. Sink the Chest and Raise the Back. "Sinking the chest" means that there is a slight drawing in of the chest allowing the *ch'i* to sink to the *tan-t'ien*. Absolutely avoid expanding the chest, for this causes the *ch'i* to be held in the chest, resulting in top-heaviness. This tends to cause a floating in the soles of the feet. "Raising the back" means that *ch'i* sticks to the back. If one is able to sink the chest, the back will naturally rise. If one is able to raise the back, then strength will issue from the back and one can overcome any opponent.

3. Relax the Waist. The waist is the ruler of the body. If the waist is relaxed, then the feet will have power and our foundation will be stable. Changes in full and empty all come from the rotation of the waist. Therefore it is said that the waist is the most vital area. If we lack power, we must look for the cause in the waist.

4. Distinguish Full and Empty. Distinguishing full and empty is the first principle in T'ai-chi ch'üan. If the weight of the whole body rests on the right leg, then the right leg is full and the left leg is empty. If the weight of the whole body rests on the left leg, then the left leg is full and the right leg is empty. Only after distinguishing full and empty will our turning movements be light, nimble and effortless. If we are not able to make this distinction, then our steps will be heavy and stiff. Our stance will be unsteady and we will be easily pulled off balance.

11

5. Sink the Shoulders and Drop the Elbows. "Sinking the shoulders" means that they are able to relax and hang downward. If they cannot be relaxed and hang downward and the shoulders are raised, then the *ch'i* rises with them and the whole body will be without power. "Dropping the elbows" means that the elbows relax and drop downward. If the elbows are pulled up, then the shoulders cannot sink. We will then not be able to push our opponents very far and will be committing the error of breaking energy as in external systems.

6. Use the Mind and Not Strength. This is stated in the "Treatise on T'ai-chi ch'üan" and means that we must rely exclusively on mind and not on strength. In practicing T'ai-chi ch'üan the whole body is relaxed. If we can eliminate even the slightest clumsiness which creates blocks in the sinews, bones and blood vessels and restricts our freedom, then our movements will be light, nimble, circular and spontaneous. Some wonder how we can be strong without using strength. The meridians of the body are like the waterways of the earth. When the waterways are open then the water flows freely; when the meridians are open then the *ch'i* passes through. If stiffness blocks the meridians, the *ch'i* and blood will be obstructed and our movements will not be nimble, then if even one hair is pulled, the whole body will be shaken. If, on the other hand, we do not use strength but use the mind, then wherever the mind goes *ch'i* will follow. In this way, if the *ch'i* flows unobstructed, daily penetrating all the passages in the entire body without interruption, then after long practice we will have achieved true internal power. This, then, is what the "Treatise on T'ai-chi ch'üan" means by "only from the highest softness comes hardness." The arms of those who have mastered T'ai-chi ch'üan are like iron concealed in cotton and are extremely heavy. When those who practice external systems are using strength it

is apparent, but when they have strength but are not applying it, then they are light and floating. It is obvious that their strength is an external, superficial kind of energy. The strength of practitioners of external systems is very easily manipulated and not worthy of praise.

7. Unity of the Upper and Lower Body. The "unity of the upper and lower body" is what the "Treatise on T'ai-chi ch'üan" means by "The root is in the feet, it is issued through the legs, controlled by the waist and expressed in the hands." From the feet to the legs to the waist there must be a continuous circuit of *ch'i* . When the hands, waist and feet move, the spirit (*shen*) of the eyes moves in unison. This, then, can be called the "unity of the upper and lower body." If just one part is not synchronized, there will be confusion.

8. The Unity of Internal and External. What T'ai-chi ch'üan trains is the spirit. Therefore it is said, "The spirit is the leader and the body is at its command." If we raise the spirit, then our movements will naturally be light and nimble. The postures are no more than full and empty, opening and closing. What we mean by opening is not limited to just the hands or feet, but we must have the idea of opening in the mind as well. What we mean by closing, too, is not limited to just the hands or feet, but we must also have the idea of closing in the mind. When the inner and outer are unified as one *ch'i* , then there is no interruption anywhere.

9. Continuity Without Interruption. The power of external stylists is extrinsic and clumsy. Therefore we see it begin and end, continue and break. The old power is exhausted before the new is born. At this level one is easily defeated by others. In T'ai-chi ch'üan we use the mind and not the strength. From beginning to end there is no interruption. Everything is complete and continuous, circular and unending. This is what the Classics

refer to as, "like a great river flowing without end," or "moving the energy like reeling silk from a cocoon." All of this expresses the idea of unity as one *ch'i*.

10. Seek Stillness In Movement. Practitioners of external systems consider leaping and crouching to be skill. They exhaust their *ch'i* and after practice are invariably out of breath. T'ai-chi uses stillness to counter movement. Even when we are moving we remain still. Therefore, in practicing the postures, the slower the better. When one slows down, then the breath becomes slow and long, the *ch'i* can sink to the *tan-t'ien* and one naturally avoids the harmful effects of elevated pulse. Students who carefully consider will be able to grasp the meaning of this.

Chapter III | Exposition of The Oral Transmission

From Cheng Man-ch'ing's *Cheng-tzu T'ai-chi ch'üan shih-san p'ien* (Master Cheng's Thirteen Chapters on T'ai-chi ch'üan), photo reprint of 1950 edition by Lan-hsi t'u-shu ch'u-pan-she, Taipei, 1975.

As a rule, martial artists who have acquired superior technique keep it secret and do not reveal it to others. It is also customary to transmit it only to sons and not to daughters. However, the sons are not always worthy and this leads to frequent loss of true transmissions. If, perhaps, a teacher has a favorite student then he will impart his technique, but always hold something back against unforseen contingencies. If we go on in this way, can one really expect to see the flowering of our national martial arts?

Although I, Man-ch'ing, studied with Master Yang Ch'eng-fu, I do not dare to claim that I received the full transmission. However, were I to hold things back, or keep secrets and not make them public, this would be to horde treasure at the expense of the nation. For the past ten or so years, whenever I desired to commit them to paper in order to spread their popularity, this feeling stirred in my mind and I put the task aside. This happened over and over, for I feared the transmission would reach the wrong people. However, after careful consideration, and in the spirit of openness and generosity, I firmly resolved to faithfully record the twelve important oral teachings in order. Master Yang did not lightly transmit these to anyone. Each time he spoke of them, he exhorted us saying, ''If I do not mention this, then even if you study for three lifetimes, it will be difficult to learn.'' If I heard these words once, I heard them a thousand times. This is how much he deeply cared, but he could not realize his great expectations. This was a cause of great pain to him. Nevertheless, I hope to provide the wise and brave men of the world with the means to study and develop, and enable all people to eliminate illness and enjoy longevity. This would be of profound benefit to the race.

1. Relaxation. Every day Master Yang repeated at least ten times: "Relax ! Relax ! Be calm. Release the whole body." Otherwise he would say, "You're not relaxed ! You're not relaxed ! Not being relaxed means that you are ready to receive a beating."

The one word, "relax," is the most difficult to achieve. All the rest follows naturally. Let me explain the main idea of Master Yang's oral instructions in order to make them readily comprehensible to students. Relaxation requires the release of all the sinews in the body without the slightest tension. This is what is known as making the waist so pliant that all of our movements appear boneless. To appear boneless means that there are only sinews. Sinews have the capacity to be released. When this is accomplished, is there any reason not to be relaxed?

2. Sinking. When we are able to completely relax, this is sinking. When the sinews release, then the body which they hold together is able to sink down.

Fundamentally, relaxation and sinking are the same thing. When one sinks, one will not float; floating is an error. If the body is able to sink, this is already very good, but we need to also sink the *ch'i*. Sinking the *ch'i* concentrates the spirit, which is enormously helpful.

3. Distinguishing Full and Empty. This is what the T'ai-chi ch'üan classics mean by, "The body in its entirety has a full and empty aspect." The right hand is connected in one line of energy with the left foot, and likewise for the left hand and right foot. If the right hand and left foot are full then the right foot and left hand are empty, and vice versa. This is what is meant by clearly distinguishing full and empty. To summarize, the weight of the body should rest on just one foot. If the weight is divided between two feet, this is double-weightedness. When turning one must take care to keep the *wei-lü* point and

the spine in alignment, in order to avoid losing central equilibrium. This is of critical importance.

4. The Light and Sensitive Energy at the Top of the Head. This means simply that the energy at the top of the head should be light and sensitive, or the idea of "holding the head as if suspended from above."

Holding the head as if suspended from above may be compared to tying one's braided hair to a rafter. The body is then suspended in mid-air not touching the ground. At this moment it is possible to rotate the entire body. If the head is independently lifted or lowered, or moved to the left or right, this will not be possible. Light and sensitive energy at the top of the head is simply the idea of suspending the head from above. This is all there is to it. When practicing the form, one should cause the *yü-chen* point at the base of the skull to stand out, then the spirit (*shen*) and *ch'i* will effortlessly meet at the top of the head.

5. The Millstone Turns But the Mind Does Not Turn. The turning of the millstone is a metaphor for the turning of the waist. The mind not turning is the central equilibrium resulting from the sinking of *ch'i* to the *tan-t'ien.*

"The millstone turns but the mind does not turn" is an oral teaching within a family transmission. It is similar to two expressions in the T'ai-chi ch'üan classics which compare the waist to an axle or a banner. This is especially noteworthy. After learning this concept, my art made rapid progress.

6. Grasp Sparrow's Tail Is Like Using a Saw. That is, the Roll-back, Ward-off, Press and Push of push-hands move back and forth like the action of a two-man saw. In using a two-man saw, each must use an equal amount of strength in order for the back and forth movement to be relaxed and without resistance. If there is the slightest

19

change on either side, the saw will become stuck at that point. If my partner causes the saw to bind, then even using strength will not draw it back, and only pushing it will free it and reestablish the balance of force. This principle has two implications for T'ai-ch ch'üan. The first is to give up oneself and follow others. By following our opponent's position we can achieve the marvelous effect of transforming energy or yielding energy. The second is that at the opponent's slightest movement, one is able to anticipate it and make the first move. That is, when the opponent seeks to throw us with a pushing force, I anticipate this by first using a pulling force. If the opponent uses a pulling force, I anticipate this by first using a pushing force.

The metaphor of the two-man saw is really an extremely profound principle. This is a true oral teaching of a family transmission and one which brought me to a kind of sudden enlightenment. Being adept at anticipating an opponent's slightest movement means that I am always in control and my opponent is always at a disadvantage. The rest goes without saying.

7. I Am Not a Meathook; Why Are You Hanging on Me? T'ai-chi ch'üan emphasizes relaxation and sensitivity and abhors stiffness and tension. If you hang your meat on meathooks, this is dead meat. How can we even discuss sensitive *ch'i*? My teacher detested and forbade this, and so scolded his students by saying that he was not a ''meathook.'' This is an oral teaching in the Yang family transmission. The concept is very profound and should be conscientiously practiced.

8. When Pushed One Does Not Topple, Like the Punching Bag Doll. The whole body is light and sensitive; the root is in the feet. If one has not mastered relaxation and sinking, this is not easily accomplished.

The punching bag doll's center of gravity is at the bottom. This is what the T'ai-chi ch'üan classics describe as. "When all the weight is sunk on one side there is freedom of movement; double-weightedness causes inflexibility." If both feet use strength at the same time, there is no doubt that one will be toppled with the first push. If there is the least stiffness or inflexibility, one will likewise be toppled with the first push. In short, the energy of the whole body, one hundred per cent of it, should be sunk on the sole of one foot. The rest of the body should be calm and lighter than a swan's down.

9. The Ability To Issue Energy. Energy and force are not the same. Energy comes from the sinews and force from the bones. Therefore, energy is a property of the soft, the alive, the flexible. Force, then, is a property of the hard, the dead and the inflexible. What do we mean by issuing energy? It is like shooting an arrow.

Shooting an arrow relies on the elasticity of the bow and string. The power of the bow and string derives from their softness, aliveness and elasticity. The difference between energy and force, the ability to issue or not issue, is readily apparent. However, this only explains the nature of issuing energy and does not fully detail its function. Allow me to add a few words on the method of issuing energy as often explained by Master Yang. He said that one must always seize the moment and gain the advantage. He also said that from the feet to the legs to the waist should be one unified flow of *ch'i.* He told us that his father, Yang Chien-hou, liked to recite these two rules. However, seizing the moment and gaining the advantage are difficult ideas to comprehend. I feel that the operation of the two-man saw contains the concept of seizing the moment and gaining the advantage. Before my opponent tries to advance or retreat, I already anticipate it. This is seizing the moment. When my opponent has already advanced or retreated, but falls under my control, this is gaining the advantage. From this example we can begin to understand that the ability to unify the feet, legs and waist into one flow of *ch'i* not only concentrates the power and gives us stamina, but prevents the body from being disunited and allows the will to be focused. The above discussion covers the marvelous effectiveness of issuing energy. Students should study this concept faithfully.

10. In Moving, Our Posture Should Be Balanced, Upright, Uniform, and Even. These four words—balanced, upright, uniform, and even—are very familiar, but very difficult to realize. Only when balanced and upright can one be comfortable and control all directions. Only when uniform and even can our movement be connected and no gaps appear. This is what the T'ai-chi classics call, "stand erect and balanced," and "energy is moved like reeling silk." If one does not begin working from these four words, it is not a true art.

11. One Must Execute Techniques Correctly. The "Song of Push-Hands" says, "In Ward-off, Roll-back, Press and Push, one must execute the correct technique." If one's knowledge is not correct, everything will become false. Let me tell you now that if in warding off, one touches the opponent's body, or if in rolling back, one allows one's own body to be touched, these are both errors. When warding off, do not touch the opponent's body; when rolling back, do not allow your own body to be touched. This is the correct technique. During Push and Press, one must reserve energy in order not to lose central equilibrium. This is correct.

I had read the words, "One must execute the correct technique," over and over in the "Classic of T'ai-chi ch'üan" without really understanding them. Only after hearing this over and over from Master Yang did I grasp the proper measure and method. Without oral instruction, it is difficult to understand. There are many such examples. This is an authentic secret teaching of a family transmission. Students should begin with this to experience it for themselves, then they can grasp the proper measure and not lose central equilibrium. This is supremely important.

12. Repelling a Thousand Pounds with Four Ounces. No one believes that four ounces can repel a thousand pounds. What is meant by ''four ounces can repel a thousand pounds'' is that only four ounces of energy need be used to pull a thousand pounds, and then the push is applied. Pulling and repelling are two different things. It is not really that one uses only four ounces to repel a thousand pounds.

By separately explaining the words, ''pull'' and ''repel,'' we can appreciate their marvelous effectiveness. The method of pulling is like putting a rope through the nose of a thousand pound bull. With a four ounce rope we can pull a thousand pound bull to the left or right as we wish. The bull is unable to escape. But the pull must be applied precisely to the nose. Pulling the horn or the leg will not work. Thus if we pull according to the correct method and at the correct point, then a bull can be pulled with only a four ounce rope. Can a thousand pound statue of a horse be pulled with a rotten rope? No! This is because of differences in the behavior of the animate and the inanimate. Human beings possess intelligence. If one attempts to attack with a thousand pounds of strength, and approaches from a certain direction, say head-on for example, then with four ounces of energy I pull his hand, and following his line of force, deflect it away. This is what we mean by pulling. After being pulled, our opponent's strength is neutralized, and at that moment I issue energy to repel him. This opponent will invariably be thrown for a great distance. The energy used to pull the opponent need only be four ounces, but the energy used to push must be adjusted to circumstances. The energy used to pull an opponent must not be too heavy, for if it is, the opponent will realize our intentions and find means of escape. Sometimes one can borrow the pulling energy, change the direction, and employ it for an attack. In other cases, the opponent realizes he is being pulled, reserves his force, and does not advance. In reserving his force, he has already put himself in a position of retreat. I can then follow his retreat, release my pulling energy, and turn to attack. The opponent is invariably toppled by our hand. This is a counter-attack.

All of the above was transmitted to me, Cheng Man-ch'ing, orally by Yang Ch'eng-fu. I do not dare keep this secret, but wish to propogate it more broadly. I sincerely hope that kindred spirits will forge ahead together.

Chapter IV

Yang Family Manuscripts Collected by Li Ying-ang

In Li Ying-ang, ed.,
T'ai-chi ch'üan shih-yung fa
(Self-defense applications of
T'ai-chi ch'üan),
Hong Kong:
Unicorn Press, 1977.

Body Principles
(attributed to Wu-Yü-hsiang, 1812-1880)

Relax the chest.
Raise the back.
Enclose the solar plexus.
Protect the cheekbones.
Lift the head.
Suspend the solar plexus.
Loosen the shoulders.
Sink the elbows.
Be evasive.
Avoid conflict.

Four Character
Secret Transmission
(attributed to Wu Yü-hsiang)

Spread. To spread means that we mobilize our *ch'i*, spread it over our opponent's energy and prevent him from moving.

Cover. To cover means that we use our *ch'i* to cover our opponent's thrust.

Check. To check means that we use *ch'i* to check our opponent's thrust, ascertain his aim, and evade it.

Swallow. To swallow means that we use *ch'i* to swallow everything and neutralize it.

These four characters represent what has no form and no sound. Without the ability to interpret energy and training to the highest perfection, they cannot be understood. We are speaking here exclusively of *ch'i*. Only if one correctly cultivates *ch'i* and does not damage it, can one project it into the limbs. The effect of this on the limbs cannot be described in words.

Songs of the Eight Ways

(attributed to T'an Meng-hsien)

The Song of Ward-off

How can we explain the energy of Ward-Off?
It is like water which supports
    a moving boat.
First make the *ch'i* in the *tan-t'ien* substantial,
Then hold the head as if suspended
    from above.
The whole body has the power of a spring.
Opening and closing should be
    clearly defined.
Even if the opponent uses a thousand pounds
    of force,
We will float lightly and without difficulty.

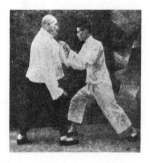

The Song of Roll-Back

How can we explain the energy of Roll-back?
We draw the opponent towards us by allowing
   him to advance,
While we follow his incoming force.
Continuing to draw him in until
   he overextends,
We remain light and comfortable,
   without losing our vertical posture.
When his force is spent
   he will naturally be empty,
While we maintain our center of gravity,
And can never be bested by the opponent.

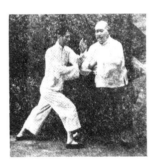

The Song of Press

How can we explain the energy of Press?
Sometimes we use two sides
To directly receive a single intention.
Meeting and combining in one movement,
We indirectly receive the force of the reaction.
This is like a ball bouncing off a wall,
Or a coin dropped on a drum,
Which bounces up with a metallic sound.

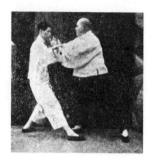

The Song of Push

How can we explain the energy of Push?
When applied, it's like water in motion
But within its softness there is great strength.
When the flow is swift, the force cannot
    be withstood.
Meeting high places the waves break over them,
And encountering low places they dive deep.
The waves rise and fall,
And finding a hole they will surely surge in.

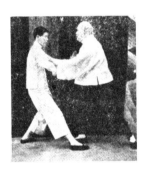

The Song of Pull-Down

How can we explain the energy of Pull-down?
Like weighing something on a balance scale,
We give free play to the opponent's force
  whether great or small.
After weighing it we know its lightness
  or heaviness.
Turning on only four ounces,
We can weigh a thousand pounds.
If we ask what is the principle behind this,
We discover it is the function of the lever.

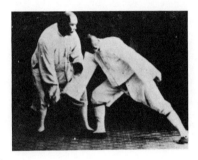

Song of Split

How can we explain the energy of Split?
Revolving like a flywheel,
If something is thrown against it,
It will be cast off at a great distance.
Whirlpools appear in swift flowing streams,
And the curling waves are like spirals.
If a falling leaf lands on their surface,
In no time it will sink from sight.

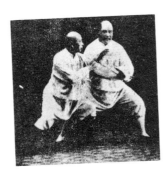

The Song of Elbow-Stroke

How can we explain the energy of
  Elbow-stroke?
Our method must be reckoned by the
  Five Elements.
Yin and *yang* are divided above and below,
And full and empty should be clearly
  distinguished.
The opponent cannot keep up with our
  continuous movement,
And our explosive pounding is even fiercer.
When the six energies have been
  thoroughly mastered,
Then the applications will be infinite.

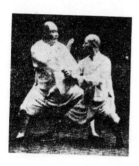

The Song of Shoulder-Stroke

How can we explain the energy of
  Shoulder-stroke?
The method is divided between shoulder
  and back.
The posture ''Diagonal Flying'' uses
  the shoulder,
But between the shoulders there is
  also the back.
When suddenly an opportunity
  presents itself,
Then it crashes like a pounding pestle.
Yet we must be careful to maintain
  our center of gravity,
For losing it we will surely fail.

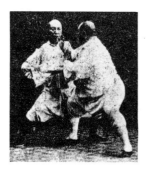

Songs of the Five Steps

Song of Advance

When it is time to advance,
  advance without hesitation.
If you meet no obstacle,
  continue to advance.
Failing to advance when the time is right
  is a lost opportunity.
Seizing the opportunity to advance,
  you will surely be the victor.

Song of Retreat

If our steps follow the changes of our body,
  then our technique will be perfect.
We must avoid fullness and emphasize
  emptiness so that our opponent lands
  on nothing.
To fail to retreat when retreat is called for
  is neither wise nor courageous.
A retreat is really an advance if
  we can turn it to a counter-attack.

Song of Gaze-Left

To the left, to the right, *yin* and *yang*
  change according to the situation.
We evade to the left and strike from the right
  with strong sure steps.
The hands and feet work together and
  likewise knees, elbows and waist.
Our opponent cannot fathom our movements
  and has no defense against us.

Song of Look-Right

Feigning to the left, we attack to the right
with perfect steps.
Striking left and attacking right,
we follow the opportunities.
We avoid the frontal and advance from the
side, seizing changing conditions.
Left and right, full and empty,
our technique must be faultless.

Song of Central Equilibrium

We are centered, stable and still
as a mountain.
Our *ch'i* sinks to the *tan-t'ien* and
we are as if suspended from above.
Our spirit is concentrated within and
our outward manner perfectly composed.
Receiving and issuing energy are
both the work of an instant.

Chapter V | # Nine Secret Transmissions on T'ai-chi ch'üan

From Wu Meng-hsia, *T'ai-chi ch'üan chiu chüeh chu-chieh* (Nine secret transmissions on T'ai-chi ch'üan with annotations), Hong Kong: T'ai-p'ing shu-chü, 1975. Author received transmissions from Niu Lien-yüan who received them from Yang Pan-hou.

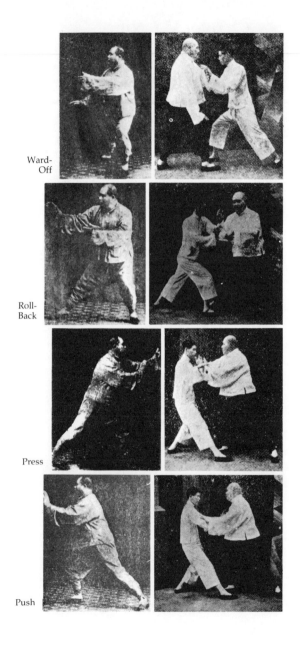

Ward-
Off

Roll-
Back

Press

Push

Secrets of T'ai-chi
Form Applications

The marvels of T'ai-chi ch'üan are infinite;
Ward-off, Roll-back, Press and Push are
   born of Grasp Sparrow's Tail.

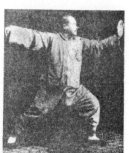

Single
Whip

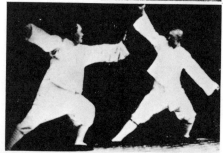

Raise
Hands

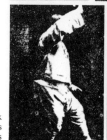

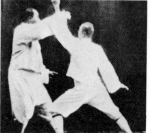

Stork
Cools
Wings

Step out on an angle and execute Single
  Whip to strike the opponent's chest;
Turn the body and perform Raise Hands
  to seal his thrust.

From Catch Moon at the Bottom of the Sea
  change to Stork Cools Wings.
Block and strike the opponent's soft
  flank without mercy.

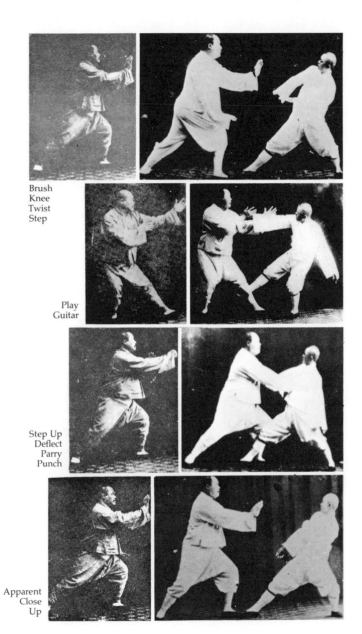

Brush
Knee
Twist
Step

Play
Guitar

Step Up
Deflect
Parry
Punch

Apparent
Close
Up

44

Brush Knee and Twist Step, seeking to
   strike him off-center;
Execute Play Guitar with perfect threading
   and transforming energy.

When sticking to the opponent's body
   and leaning close, use the elbows to
   strike horizontally;
If the elbow is caught, circle back and
   strike with the fist for equal success.

Step Up, Deflect, Parry and Punch the ribs;
Use Apparent Close Up to protect the center.

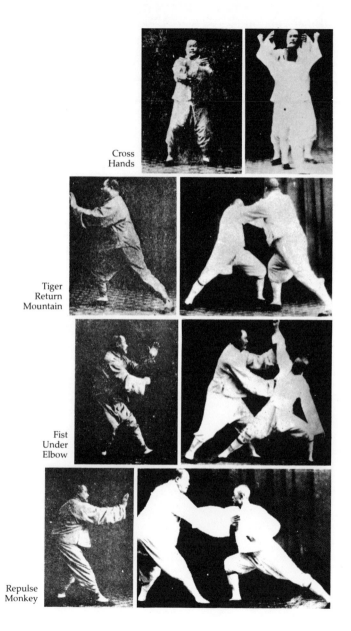

Cross
Hands

Tiger
Return
Mountain

Fist
Under
Elbow

Repulse
Monkey

The permutations of Cross Hands are infinite;
Embrace Tiger Return to Mountain
   demonstrates Pull-down and Split.

Fist Under Elbow protects the middle joint;
Take three steps back for Repulse Monkey.

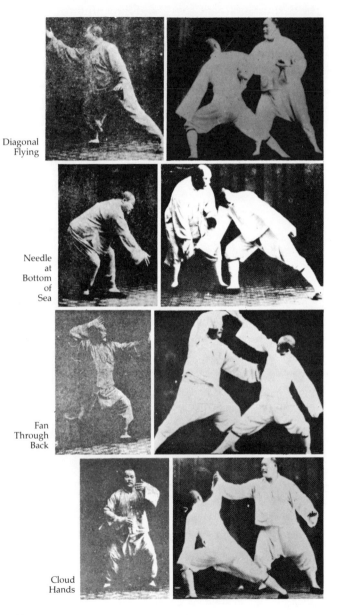

Diagonal Flying

Needle at Bottom of Sea

Fan Through Back

Cloud Hands

48

Sink the body when retreating and use
    the pulling power of the wrist;
The technique of Diagonal Flying is
    infinitely useful.

For Needle at the Bottom of the Sea
    we must bend the body down;
Fan Through the Back employs the skill
    of bracketing.

The method for breaking locks lies in
    the wrist;
Advance three times with Cloud Hands,
    demonstrating skill with the top of
    the forearm.

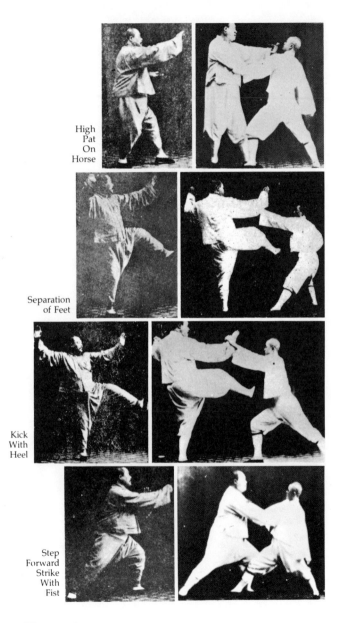

High
Pat
On
Horse

Separation
of Feet

Kick
With
Heel

Step
Forward
Strike
With
Fist

50

High Pat on Horse is used to block and stab;
For Left and Right Separation of the Feet
   we must first grasp the opponent's wrist.

Use Turn and Kick with Heel to Strike
   the opponent's abdomen;
Execute Step Forward and Strike with
   Fist to directly attack his face.

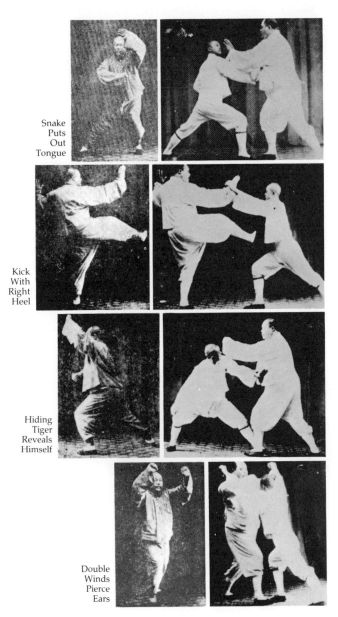

Snake
Puts
Out
Tongue

Kick
With
Right
Heel

Hiding
Tiger
Reveals
Himself

Double
Winds
Pierce
Ears

52

Turn the body and change to White
Snake Puts Out Tongue;
Grasp the opponent's hand and strike
the eyes.

Direct Kick with Right Heel to the
opponent's soft flank;
Perfectly execute Hiding Tiger Reveals
Himself to the left and right.

Come up and strike the opponent's breast
and below the ribs;
The technique of Double Winds Pierce
the Ears is most effective.

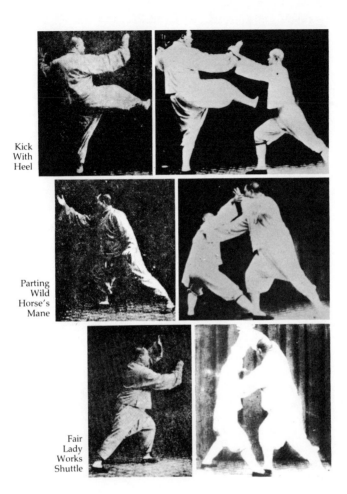

Kick
With
Heel

Parting
Wild
Horse's
Mane

Fair
Lady
Works
Shuttle

54

Kick Left with Heel is the same as
  Kick Right with Heel;
Use Turn the Body and Kick, aiming for
  the knee.

Parting the Wild Horse's Mane is used
  to attack below the armpit;
Fair Lady Works Shuttles seals the
  four corners.

Use Fair Lady to remove the opponent's
  arm and elevate it;
Left and right, the application is the same.

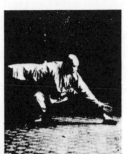

Squatting
Single
Whip

Golden
Cock
Stands
On One
Leg

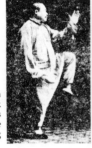

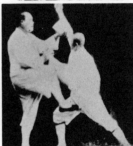

Squatting Single Whip follows the
   fingertips to invade the opponent's
   private parts;
Golden Cock Stands on One Leg gives
   one absolute sway.

Raise the knee and strike the most
   vital organ;
Or use the other leg to trample the
   opponent's feet without mercy.

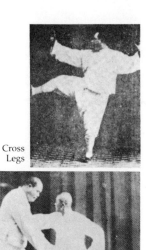

Cross
Legs

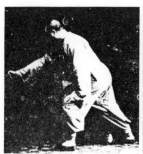

Punch
The
Crotch

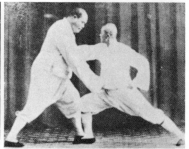

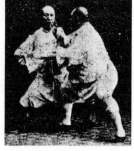

Shoulder
Stroke

58

The technique of Cross Legs breaks
    the soft bone below the knee;
If Punch the Crotch is not successful,
    follow up with a Shoulder-stroke.

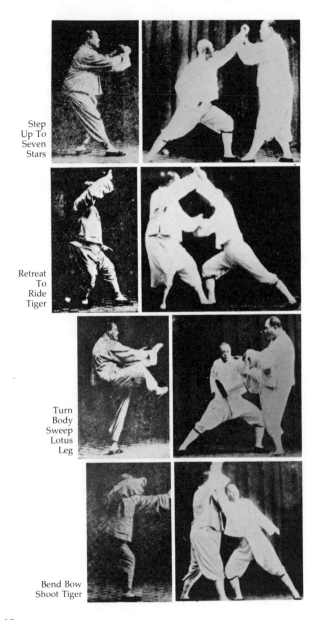

Step
Up To
Seven
Stars

Retreat
To
Ride
Tiger

Turn
Body
Sweep
Lotus
Leg

Bend Bow
Shoot Tiger

The posture Step Up to Seven Stars forms
  a rack with the hands;
Retreat to Ride Tiger swiftly withdraws
  our center.

When executing Turn Body Sweep Lotus Leg,
  make certain to protect the advancing leg;
Use Bend Bow and Shoot Tiger to strike
  the opponent's chest.

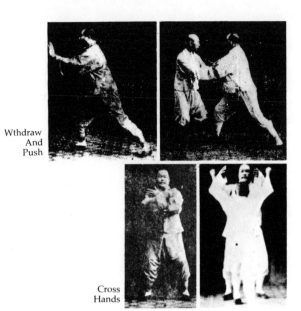

Wthdraw
And
Push

Cross
Hands

62

During Withdraw and Push be attentive to
   Gaze-left, Look-right and Central
   Equilibrium;
Cross Hands closes the T'ai-chi form.

In practicing form applications, the most
   important thing is the mind;
Relax the body, stabilize the *ch'i* and
   concentrate the spirit.

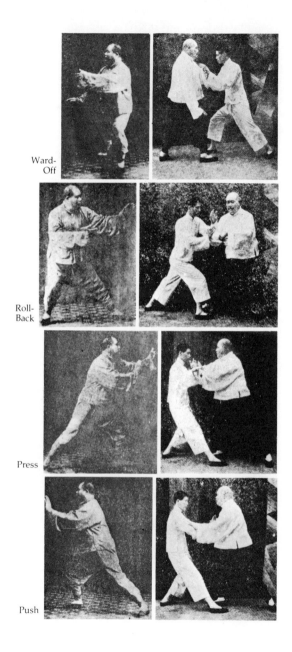

Ward-
Off

Roll-
Back

Press

Push

Secrets of the Applications
of the Thirteen Postures

In Ward-off, the two arms should be
   rounded and as if propped up;
Whether active or still, empty or full,
   the potential for attack is always there.

When hands are joined with the opponent,
   first Roll-back and then use Press;
If the opponent wishes to counter,
   it will prove most difficult.

In applying Push, it looks as if we
   might topple;
Make contact at two points and
   do not release them.

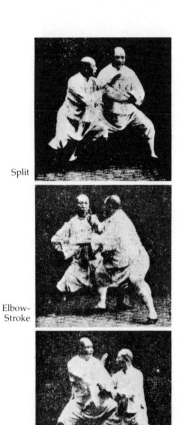

Split

Elbow-
Stroke

Shoulder-
Stroke

When the attack is fierce, use the
technique Split;
Elbow-stroke and Shoulder-stroke can
be applied when opportunities arise

Advancing, retreating, turning around
or sideways, we move in response to
conditions;
What fear have we of an opponent's
excellent technique?

When confronting an opponent do
not be afraid to close with him,
But be careful of one's own Three Forwards
[hands, feet and eyes]
and the opponent's Seven Stars
[shoulders, elbows, knees, hips,
head, hands and feet].

When an opponent closes with us
forcefully and strikes,
We must quickly evade by withdrawing
our center and attacking from the side.

The methods embodied in T'ai-chi's
Thirteen Postures,
Must be faithfully practiced and then
their marvels will unfold.

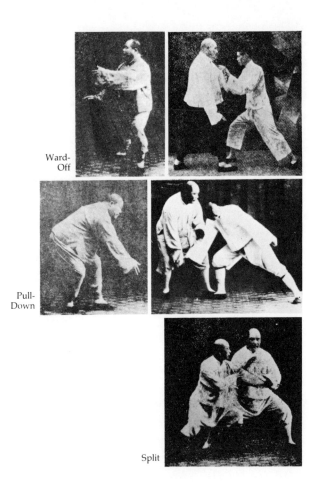

Ward-
Off

Pull-
Down

Split

Secrets of the Use of the Thirteen Postures

If we meet an opponent whose Ward-off
  does not allow us to penetrate the circle,
By simply sticking and adhering it will
  be difficult for us to make headway.

If we are sealed off by our opponent's
  Ward-off, then we must try Pull-down
  or split;
If these are successful, capitalize
  immediately and without delay.

I control my own four sides and seek
  gaps in my opponent's four corners;
After contact is made, whoever acts
  effectively first will prevail.

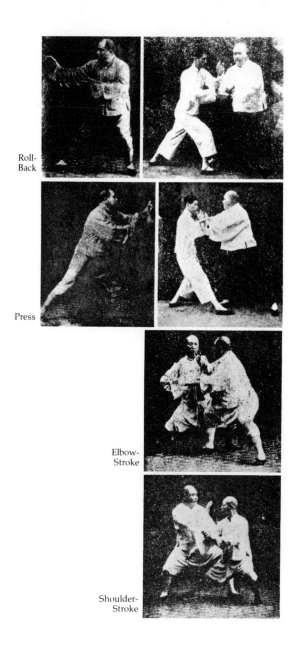

Roll-
Back

Press

Elbow-
Stroke

Shoulder-
Stroke

The two methods, Roll-back and Press,
   should be used at the right opportunity;
When applying Elbow-stroke and Shoulder-
   stroke place yourself before the
   opponent's heel.

Advance and retreat as the situation
   calls for;
Use Gaze-left and Look-right always mindful
   of the Three Forwards and Seven Stars.

The real power of the whole body should
   be concentrated in the center;
Listening, interpreting, following and
   neutralizing must be imbued with spirit
   and *ch'i*.

If we see a solid opportunity and fail
   to take advantage of it,
How can it be said that our art is complete?

If we do not practice according to the
   applications of the principles,
We can work forever without developing
   a superior art.

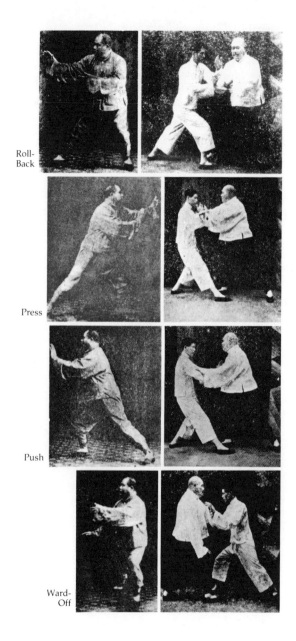

Roll-
Back

Press

Push

Ward-
Off

Secrets of the
Eight Word Method

During Push-hands, there are three
   exchanges, including two Roll-backs
   and one Press and Push.
When hands are joined and we encounter
   Ward-off, do not let the opponent
   get the upper hand.

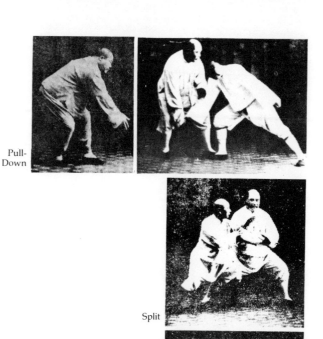

Pull-
Down

Split

Elbow-
Stroke

If there is hardness within our softness,
    we will never be defeated,
But if our hardness does not contain softness,
    it cannot be called firm.

In order to break an opponent's offense
    or defense, use Pull-down or Split;
Put power into a surprise thrust or
    quick rotation.

If an opening appears and we have already
    closed with the opponent, then use
    Elbow-stroke;
To strike with shoulders, hips or
    knees we first draw very near.

**The Secret of
Full and Empty**

Empty empty, full full, with spirit
    ever present;
Empty full, full empty as hands
    perform techniques.

To practice T'ai-chi without mastering
    the principle of full and empty,
Is to foolishly waste time without ever
    accomplishing anything.

When one has the opponent's vital point
    in the palm of one's hand; finding empty,
    be on guard, but if full, attack.
If we fail to attack the full,
    our art will never be superior.

Within empty and full, there is
    naturally a full and empty;
If we understand the principle of full and
    empty, our attack will never miss the mark.

The Secret of the Free Circle

The technique of the free circle is
   most difficult to master;
Up, down, following and joining,
   it is infinitely marvelous.

If we can entice the opponent into
   our circle,
Then the technique of four ounces repelling
   a thousand pounds will succeed.

When the maximum power of the hands
   and feet arrives together seeking a
   straight line to the side,
Then our advantage from the free circle
   will not be wasted.

If we desire to know the method of the circle,
We must first find the correct point to issue
   from and the correct target,
   and then we will accomplish our task.

The Secret of *Yin* and *yang*

Few have truly cultivated the *yin* and *yang*
   of T'ai-chi;
Swallowing and spitting, opening and closing
   give expression to hard and soft.

Controlling the cardinal directions and corners,
   drawing in and issuing forth,
   let the opponent do what he will;
All is but the transformations of action and
   stillness, so what need is there to worry?

Offense and defense must be intimately
   coordinated;
Evading and attacking must be sought
   in every action.

What is the meaning of light and heavy,
   full and empty?
As soon as we discover lightness within
   our opponent's heaviness, we must
   attack without hesitation.

The Secrets of the Eighteen Loci

Ward-off is in the two arms.
Roll-back is in the palms.
Press is in the back of the hand.
Push is in the waist.
Pull-down is in the fingers.
Split is in the two forearms.
Elbow-stroke involves bending the limbs.
Shoulder-stroke employs shoulder against chest.
Advancing is found in Cloud Hands.
Retreating is found in Repulse Monkey.
Gaze-left is in the Three Forwards.
Look-right is in the Seven Stars.
Stability involves waiting for an opportunity.
The bull's-eye is reached by attacking
   from the side.
Clumsiness results from double-weightedness.
Agility derives from single lightness.
Emptiness means not attacking.
Fullness means attacking.

Secrets of the Five Character Classic

Exposure means to attack from the
 opponent's side.
Evading and turning aside must not be
 completely empty.
Neutralize the opponent's incoming force
 with outstretched arms.
Use tentative give and take to test
 the opponent's skill.
Reserve your power and concentrate it for
 the right moment.
Sticking and adhering are our guiding
 principles.
Move as if following, whether advancing
 or retreating.
Never forget the possibility of capturing
 the opponent's hand.
Use strangle holds to block the
 opponent's circulation.
If the opponent seeks to twist or lock our hands,
 follow his incoming force and block him.
The meaning of softness is that we do not use
 stiff force.
In Ward-off the arms should be rounded
 and look as if propped up.
Pull and attack with circular and lively power.
We must blunt our opponent's sharp thrusts,
Protect ourselves from his fierce penetration,
And use the finger to stab his vital points.
We must use sinking to escape from
 pulling or twisting of our wrist.
Continue to follow without allowing gaps.
When we use Press our opponent's
 full and empty will appear;
Apply repelling force and victory
 is quickly ours.

Chapter VI | Yang Family Manuscripts Copied by Shen Chia-chen

In T'ang Hao and Ku Liu-hsing,
T'ai-chi ch'üan yen-chiu
(Studies on T'ai-chi ch'üan).
Hong Kong:
Pai-ling ch'u-pan-she, n.d.

The Meaning of Leveling the Waist and Crown of the Head in T'ai-chi

The crown of the head should be level, therefore it is said that "the top of the head should be as if suspended from above." The two hands travel in orbits left and right, while the waist is the root. If we stand level and maintain this in the body, then we will be able to detect the minutest degrees of lightness or heaviness, floating or sinking. Expressing the idea of levelness as if suspended from above (meaning one straight line from the crown of the head down through the root of the waist and from the *hsiung-men* point in the middle of the back to the *wei-lü* point at the base of the spine) there is a song that goes:

One straight line from top to bottom;
All depends upon the turning of the hands.
Changes are gauged by the slightest degree,
Clearly distinguishing feet and inches.
The waist is like a cartwheel,
Which turns when the streamers unfurl.
The mind commands and the *ch'i* goes into
   action like banners.
I move naturally, following my own convenience.
My whole body is light and agile,
Tempered like a diamond arhat.
My opponent weaves in and out,
But sooner or later,
We will make contact and he will be repelled,
Even without my unleashing a mighty thunderbolt.
We must know how long to dally,
And how to make them faint with a shout.
This oral teaching must be transmitted secretly.
Open the gate and behold, this is truly Heaven!

The Meaning of T'ai-chi's
Proper Functioning

T'ai-chi, in its round aspect, whether moving in or out, up or down, left or right never leaves the circle. T'ai-chi, in its square aspect, whether in or out, up or down, left or right never leaves the square. The circle is for issuing or entering; the square is for advancing or retreating. There is a constant back and forth movement from the square to the circle. The square is for opening and expanding and the circle is for closing and contracting.

When one has mastered the law of the circle and the square, how can there be anything beyond it? This is grasped with the mind and reflected in the hands. Gaze up at the heights and bore deeper and deeper. It is marvelous and ever more marvelous. It is concealed in the subtle, brighter and brighter, growing and growing without end. We cannot stop even if we wished to.

The Meaning of Light and Heavy,
Floating and Sinking in T'ai-chi

1. Double weightedness is an error. The error lies in misplaced fullness and is not the same as sinking.

2. Double sinking is not an error, but natural buoyancy and emptiness. It is not the same thing as weightedness.

3. Double floating is an error, for it is drifting and vague. It should not be confused with lightness.

4. Double lightness is not an error, for it is naturally light and sensitive. It has nothing in common with floating. Half light and half heavy is not an error. "Half" means that one is half settled and therefore it is not an error. Partially light and partially heavy is an error. "Partially" means that one is not settled and therefore it is an error. When one is not settled, the square and the circle will be lost. When one is half settled, how can this be considered leaving the square and the circle?

84

5. Half floating and half sinking is an error. The fault lies in insufficiency.

6. Partial floating and partial sinking is an error. The fault lies in excess.

7. Half heavy and partially heavy is an error, for it is stiff and incorrect.

8. Half light and partially light is an error. It is sensitive but not circular.

9. Half sinking and partial sinking is an error, for it is empty and incorrect.

10. Half floating and partial floating is an error, for it is vague and not circular.

11. Double lightness is not the same as floating, for it is light and sensitive. If double lightness does not become floating, then it is light and sensitive; if double sinking does not become heavy, then it becomes open and empty. Therefore it is said that the superior practitioner is light and heavy; those who are half settled are merely common practitioners. Aside from these three, all of the rest are erroneous techniques. When one is empty, sensitive and clear within, it will naturally express itself without. When there is clarity in the body, it will flow into the four limbs. If one fails to thoroughly study the four qualities—light, heavy, floating and sinking—it will be as frustrating as digging a well without reaching the spring. One whose technique encompasses the square, the circle and the four cardinal points and has mastered the internal, external, fine and gross has already achieved much. Why should we worry about something arising from the four corners to confound our square and circle? So it is said, ''from the square to the circle and the circle to the square.'' The superior practitioner achieves a realm beyond phenomena.

The Meaning of Strength Versus
Ch'i in T'ai-chi

Ch'i runs in the channels of the internal membranes and sinews. Strength issues from the blood, flesh, skin and bones. Thus those possessed of strength are externally sturdy in their skin and bones, that is, in their physical form; those possessed of *ch'i* have internal strength in their sinews, that is, their charisma (*hsiang*). *Ch'i* and blood work to strengthen the internal; the *ch'i* of the blood works to strengthen the external.

In summary, if you understand the function of the two words—*ch'i* and blood—then you will naturally know the origin of strength and *ch'i*. If you know the nature of strength and *ch'i*, you will know the difference between using strength and mobilizing *ch'i*. Mobilizing *ch'i* in the sinews and using strength in the skin and bones are two vastly different things.

The Meaning of Civil and Martial in T'ai-chi

The civil is the essence and the martial is the function. When civil attainments are actively applied through martial arts in the form of vital energy (*ching*), *ch'i*, and spirit (*shen*), this is called the essence of the civil. When martial attainments are accompanied by the essence of the civil in the mind and the body, this is called martial practice. The civil and the martial are also called the art of self-cultivation.

When yielding and repelling are correctly timed, then the root of the essence of the civil, that is, martial practice executed according to civil principle, belongs to the soft essence of the civil. When storing and issuing are applied at the appropriate time, then the root of martial practice, that is, the civil applied through martial practice, belongs to the category of hard martial practice. Vital energy, *ch'i* and spirit and the sinews and bones are the civil and the martial. Hard martial practice is simply muscular force. However, to have the civil without martial preparation is the essence without the function; to have the martial which is not coupled with the civil is the function without the essence.

A single wooden board cannot support a whole structure; a single hand cannot make a clapping sound. This is not only true of civil essence and martial practice, but of all things in the world. The civil is the inner principle and the martial is the outer technique. Outer technique without inner principle is simply the brute courage of physical strength. However, when one is no longer in the prime, bullying an opponent will not work. Those who possess inner principle without outer technique, who think only of the arts of quietism and know nothing of the practice of combat, are lost as soon as they commit the slightest error. Whether for practical pursuits or simply the way of being a human being, how dare we neglect the two words—civil and martial?

The Meaning of Stick, Adhere, Join and Follow

Raising up and lifting high
   is called sticking.
Attachment and inseparability
   is called adhering.
Forgetting oneself and not separating from
   the opponent is called joining.
Responding to the opponent's every
   movement is called following.

If we wish to understand conscious movement, it is essential to be clear about sticking, adhering, joining and following. This skill is extremely subtle.

The Meaning of Butting, Thinness, Losing and Resistance

Butting means over-extending the head.
Thinness means an insufficiency.
Losing means separation.
Resistance means an excess.

We must understand the errors represented by these four words. Not only will they impede our cultivation of sticking, adhering, joining and following, but will also cloud our understanding of conscious movement. Beginners in self-defense must strive to understand this and make special efforts to avoid these four errors. What is difficult about sticking, adhering, joining and following is that we must not commit the errors of butting, thinness, losing or resistance. This is why it is not easy.

Self-Defense Without Errors

Butting, thinness, losing and resistance are failures in self-defense. That is why they are called errors. When one has failed to stick, adhere, join and follow, how can one hope for conscious movement? Since one is not even aware of this oneself, how can one know it in others? What we mean by self-defense without errors is not being guilty of butting, thinness, losing and resistance in dealing with an opponent. Rather, we use sticking, adhering, joining and following. If we are successful in this, we will not only be free of error, but will naturally achieve conscious movement and advance to the ability to interpret energy.

The Song of Holding the Center
in Self-Defense Training

The feet must be rooted in the posture
    Central Equilibrium.
First understand the four cardinal directions,
    advance and retreat.
Ward-off, Roll-back, Press and Push
    require four hands to practice,
And a great deal of effort must be expended
    to grasp their true significance.
The body, form, waist and crown of the head
    must all be brought into play.
In sticking, adhering, joining and following,
    the mind and *ch'i* are rulers.
The spirit is the ruler and the flesh
    and bones are subjects.
Clearly understanding all aspects
    of our art,
We will naturally achieve perfection
    in the martial and the civil.

Song of the T'ai-chi Circle

The circle of retreat is easy;
    the circle of advance is difficult.
Do not deviate from the correct position of the
    waist or crown of the head,
    whether to the rear or fore.
What is most difficult is not deviating
    from Central Equilibrium.
Carefully consider the principle that to
    retreat is easy but to advance is difficult.
This has to do with the art of movement
    and not with static postures.

We must advance and retreat while keeping
   shoulder to shoulder with our opponent.
Be like the millstone moving fast or slow,
Or whirling like the Cloud Dragon
   or Wind Tiger.
Begin your search with the aid of compass,
And after a long time it will become
   perfectly natural.

The Meaning of Four Corners in T'ai-chi ch'üan

The four cardinal directions refer to the four sides of the square, or Ward-off, Roll-back, Press and Push. Before understanding that the square can be made round and the principle of the infinite alternating squares and circles, how can one expect to master the techniques of the four corners? Because of man's four members without and spirit within, it is most difficult to acquire mastery of the square, the circle and the four cardinal directions. However, when one begins to commit errors of lightness and heaviness, floating and sinking, then the four corners come into play. For example, if because of half or partial weightedness one's movements are clumsy and incorrect, then one will naturally execute the four-corner techniques: Pull-down, Split, Elbow-stroke and Shoulder-stroke. Or, if one is guilty of double-weightedness, then likewise four-corner techniques will appear.

With erroneous technique, one has no choice but to use the four corners to help return to the framework of squareness and roundness. Thus Pull-down, Split, Elbow-stroke and Shoulder-stroke make up for deficiencies. Those who after long practice have reached a high level of skill must also acquire Pull-down and Split to return everything to center. In this way the four corners have a supplementary function and compensate for deficiencies.

The Meaning of the Martial Aspect of T'ai-chi

T'ai-chi in its martial aspect is soft on the outside and hard on the inside. If we constantly seek to be soft on the outside, after a long time we will naturally attain hardness on the inside. It is not that we deliberately think of hardness, for in reality our minds are on softness. The difficulty lies in being hard within but restraining its expression externally. We must at all times use softness to meet the opponent, that is, meet hardness with softness and reduce hardness to nothing. How can this be achieved? Briefly, having mastered sticking, adhering, joining and following, and after understanding conscious movement, one can progress to interpreting energy. After learning to interpret energy, one naturally arrives by stages at the level of highest perfection. In the end, we will complete our task and reach the goal.

As for the marvel of four ounces repelling a thousand pounds, how could this be possible if one's skill has not yet reached the supreme? Therefore, only after one understands sticking, adhering, joining and following can one acquire the skills of seeing, hearing, lightness and sensitivity.

Treatise on Before and After Acquiring the Ability to Interpret Energy in T'ai-chi

Before being able to interpret energy one is often guilty of errors of butting, thinness, losing and resistance. After being able to interpret energy, there is still a possibilty of committing errors associated with stooping, rising, breaking and continuity. Before one can interpret energy there will naturally be faulty technique, but after one can interpret energy, how could this still persist? When one is at the stage of seeming to interpret energy but not yet interpreting properly, that is, in a state of ambivalence, then one's breaking and contacting will be inaccurate and there will be many errors. Before one has reached the highest perfection, stooping and rising will miss the mark and it will be easy to make errors. If one has not mastered breaking, contacting, stooping and rising, and does not truly understand interpreting energy, then these errors are unavoidable.

Therefore, those who do not yet truly understand interpreting energy, because their seeing and hearing are without basis, have not yet achieved precision. Only when one understands the visual awareness of looking far, near, left and right; the aural awareness of rising falling, slowness and haste; the kinesthetic awareness of dodge, return, provoke and finish; and the movement awareness of turn, exchange, advance and retreat, can one truly be said to have mastered interpreting energy.

After being capable of interpreting energy, one will naturally arrive by degrees at the highest perfection. One will naturally possess superiority in withdrawing, extending, advancing and retreating, for, in this way, withdrawing, extending, movement, stillness, opening, closing, rising and falling will all have a foundation. On the basis of withdrawing, extending, movement and stillness, when one sees entering then one opens, when one meets issuing then one closes, when one observes coming then one lowers, and when one sees the opponent fleeing then one rises. After all this, then and only then can one truly reach the highest perfection. Understanding this, how can one not be prudent in regard to such habits as sitting, sleeping, walking, standing, drinking, eating, urination and defecation in order to promote the best results? In this way we can progress to medium and great accomplishments.

The Meaning of Feet, Inches, Hundredth Parts and Thousandth Parts in T'ai-chi

In the martial arts we first learn opening and expanding and then later contracting and gathering. Only after having mastered opening and expanding can one begin to discuss contracting and gathering. After contracting and gathering have been mastered, we can begin to discuss feet, inches, hundredth parts and thousandth parts. When one has mastered feet, one can begin to make divisions by the unit of the inch; when one has mastered inches one can make divisions by hundredth parts, and when the hundredth parts unit is mastered, then one makes divisions by thousandth parts. This then clarifies what is meant by feet, inches, hundredth parts and thousandth parts.

There are ten [Chinese] inches to the foot, ten hundredth parts to the inch, and ten thousandth parts to the hundredth part, so there is a definite number. There is an ancient saying that self-defense is a matter of numbers. If one understands the concept of number, one can ascertain the feet, inches, hundredth and thousandth parts. However, although we may understand the numbers, without secret transmissions, how would we be able to measure them?

Chapter VII

From Yang Ch'eng-fu's
Self-Defense Applications of T'ai-chi ch'üan

Yang Ch'eng-fu, *T'ai-chi ch'üan shih-yung fa* (Self-defense applications of T'ai-chi ch'üan), Taipei: Chung-hua wu-shu ch'u-pan-she, 1974 (first edition, 1931); also in Sung Shih-yüan, *T'ai-chi ch'üan yün-chen t'u-chieh* (The true principles of T'ai-chi ch'üan illustrated and explained), Taipei: Hua-lien ch'u-pan-she, 1967; and Yang Ch'eng-fu, *T'ai-chi ch'üan yung-fa t'u-chieh* (Applications of T'ai-chi ch'üan illustrated and explained), Taipei: Hua-lien ch'u-pan-she, 1980.

T'ai-chi Symbol

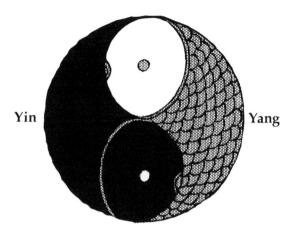

Yin   **Yang**

The meaning of the T'ai-chi symbol lies in the mutual production of *yin* and *yang*, the complementary exchange of hard and soft, the thousand changes and ten thousand transformations. This is the basis for T'ai-chi ch'üan. Push-hands is the embodiment of the T'ai chi symbol.

Original Introduction to T'ai-chi ch'üan

T'ai-chi ch'üan was handed down by the Immortal, Chang San-feng. The Immortal was a native of I-chou in Liaotung Province. His Taoist style was San-feng and he was born during the latter part of the Sung dynasty (960—1126). He was seven feet tall with the bones of a crane and the posture of a pine tree. His face was like an ancient moon with kind brows and generous eyes. His whiskers were shaped like a spear and in winter and summer he wore the same wide bamboo hat. Carrying a horsehair duster he could cover a thousand miles in a day.

During the beginning of the Hung-wu reign [first emperor, T'ai Tsu, of the Ming, 1368—1628] He traveled to the T'ai-ho Mountains in Szechwan to practice the Taoist arts and settled in the Temple of the Jade Void. He could recite the Classics by heart after a single reading. In the twenty-seventh year of the Hung-wu reign he traveled to the Wutang Mountains in Hupei where he loved to discuss the Classics and philosophy with the local people.

One day he was indoors reciting the Classics when a joyful bird landed in the courtyard. Its song was like the notes of the zither. The Immortal spied the bird from his window. The bird peered down like an eagle at a snake coiled on the ground. The snake gazed up at the bird and the two commenced to fight. With a cry the bird swooped down, spreading its wings and beating like a fan. The long snake shook its head, darting hither and thither to evade the bird's wings. The bird flew back up to the tree top, very frustrated and disconcerted. Again the bird swooped down beating with its wings, and again the snake wriggled and darted out of harm's way, all from a coiled position. This went on for a long time without a decisive strike.

After a time the Immortal came out and the bird and the snake disappeared. From this combat the Immortal received a revelation. The coiled form was like the symbol of T'ai-chi and contained the principle of the soft overcoming the hard. Based on the transformations of T'ai-chi [the Great Ultimate] he developed T'ai-chi ch'üan to cultivate sexual energy (*ching*), *ch'i* and spirit (*shen*), movement and stillness, waxing and waning and to embody the principles of the *I ching*. It has been passed on for many generations and its value has become more and more appreciated. In the White Cloud Temple at Peking there is still a likeness of the Immortal for visitors to admire.

A Story of Yang Lu-ch'an

When Master went to the capital, Peking, his fame spread far and wide. There was a constant stream of martial artists coming to pay their respects. One day, while he was sitting in meditation, a monk arrived unannounced and Master went to the steps to greet him. He noticed that the monk was powerfully built and more than six feet tall. The monk saluted and expressed his great admiration. Master was about to humbly reply when the monk flew at him, attacking with his fists. Master slightly depressed his chest and with his right palm patted the monk's fist. As if struck by a bolt of lightning, the monk was thrown behind a screen, his body still in the attitude of attacking with clenched fists. After a long time the monk, looking very solemn, apologized saying, ''I have been extremely rude.''

Master Yang invited the monk to stay for a chat and learned that his name was Ch'ing-te and that he was a Shaolin boxer. The monk plied him with endless questions. He asked, ''Just a moment ago why was I surprised and unable to display my prowess?'' Master responded, ''This is because I am always on my guard.''

The monk then asked, "How were you able to react so quickly?" Master said, "This is called issuing energy like shooting an arrow." The monk replied, "I have roamed over many provinces, but have never met your equal, Sir. I beg you to teach me the secret of T'ai-chi's lightness and sensitivity."

Master did not respond to the monk's last question but saw a sparrow fly in through the curtain and circle down close to him. He quickly caught the bird in his hand and said to the monk, "This bird is very tame and I'm going to have a little fun with it." He placed it on the palm of his right hand and stroked it gently with his left. Then he removed his left hand altogether and the sparrow beat its wings and attempted to take off. Master used the technique of "suddenly concealing and suddenly revealing" and the sparrow was unable to fly away. This is because regardless of the species of bird all must first apply energy with the feet in order to lift into flight. The sparrow's feet were unable to find a place to exert pressure and it gradually settled down. Master again stroked it and released it, but again it could not take off. After the third time, the monk, greatly amazed, exclaimed, "Your art is truly miraculous!" Master laughed and said, "This hardly deserves to be called miraculous. If one practices T'ai-chi for some time, the entire body becomes so light and sensitive that a feather weight cannot be added without setting it into motion and a fly cannot alight without the same effect. This is all there is to it." The monk bowed deeply, stayed for three days and then departed.

Yang Lu-ch'an's
Commentary to the T'ai-chi ch'üan Classic

This is a transmission of Master Chang San-feng of the Wutang Mountains. He desired longevity for all the worthy men of the world and not simply that they practice the superficial techniques of the martial arts.

As soon as one moves, the entire body should be light and sensitive and all its parts connected.

When practicing the form do not use clumsy force and you will be able to achieve lightness and sensitivity. The entire form should be performed with one continuous flow of *ch'i.*

The Ch'i should be roused and the spirit gathered within.

If the *ch'i* is not blocked it is like a sea wind which blows up waves and billows. Still the mind and concentrate the spirit. This is what is meant by gathering the spirit within.

Do not allow gaps; do not allow bulges or hollows; do not allow discontinuities.

When doing the form seek perfect wholeness. There should not be the slightest irregularity. You should move slowly and without breaks.

The root is in the feet, energy issues up through the legs, is controlled by the waist and is expressed in the hands and fingers. From the feet to the legs to the waist should be one complete flow of ch'i. One will then be able to seize opportunities and occupy the superior position.

When practicing T'ai-chi ch'üan, the upper and lower parts of the body must be coordinated. Intrinsic power (*chin*) rises from the soles of the feet, travels up the legs and reaches the waist. Then from the spine to the shoulders it travels into the hands and fingers. The whole body is as one *ch'i*. When it is used to advance or retreat, the intrinsic power is infinite.

If one is unable to seize opportunities and gain the superior position, the body will be scattered and in confusion. Look for the weakness in the waist and the legs. The same is true for above and below, front and back, left and right. All of this has to do with the mind and not with externals.

The weakness is not in externals but in the mental attitude. If the mind is not focused, then the spirit will not be concentrated and one will not be able to seize opportunities and gain the superior position.

If there is an above, there must be a below; if there is a fore, there must be a rear and if there is a left, there must be a right. If the intention is to rise one must pay attention to below. If you want to lift something, you must apply breaking power. In this way its root will be severed and its destruction will be swift and inevitable.

This means that when sparring with an opponent you must first shake him and cause him to be like a tree without roots. When his stance is not stable he will surely be toppled.

Full and Empty should be clearly distinguished. Any given point has the potential for full or empty and the whole body has this dual aspect: full and empty.

When sparring with an opponent, every posture should be full in front and empty behind. When issuing energy the front leg bears the weight of the body and is full, while the rear leg is straight. Always clearly distinguish full and empty and you will naturally have the ability to change at will.

All the joints of the body should be connected without permitting the slightest break.

All the joints of the body should be pliant and unified. The *ch'i* should flow unimpeded and there should be no breaks in consciousness .

An Explanation of the Macrocosmic and Microcosmic T'ai-chi

The whole universe is one great T'ai-chi; the human body is a small T'ai-chi. The human body being the essence of T'ai-chi, one cannot but practice the Great Ultimate Martial Art [T'ai-chi ch'üan]. It is an inborn sensitivity which must be retrained, an innate ability.

The human body is like a machine. If it is not polished for a long time it rusts. When there is ''rust'' the *ch'i* and the blood are obstructed and many faults appear. Therefore, if men desire to discipline their bodies, they should first practice T'ai-chi, for this is the most suitable means.

The method of training in T'ai-chi consists of moving the *ch'i* with the mind and not using clumsy force. Allow everything to be completely natural. The sinews and bones experience very little of the pain of bending and the skin none of the hardship of rough contact.

If we do not use strength, how can we be strong? In the art of T'ai-chi we sink the shoulders and drop the elbows. By sinking the *ch'i* to the *tan-t'ien* the *ch'i* is able to enter the *tan-t'ien* which becomes its central headquarters. From here it can be mobilized to the four limbs and hundred bones. When the *ch'i* circulates throughout the entire body, then wherever the mind goes the *ch'i* will follow. When you reach this level your power will be immeasurable.

Thus without using clumsy force and relying purely on spirit to move, the results are tremendous. My master said, "Only from great softness comes great hardness." This is my meaning.

An Explanation of
Wang Tsung-yüeh's Original Introduction

By moving the ch'i with the mind and directing it to sink, it is able to permeate the bones.

Normally during our practice of the Thirteen Postures we should use the mind to cause the *ch'i* to circulate in the space between the bones and the flesh. If the mind acts as guide, the *ch'i* will follow. As for our postures, they should be sunk and open. Our mental attitude should be calm. Without a calm mind there can be no sinking and without sinking the *ch'i* will not gather in the bones. One may indeed possess external power, but by practicing T'ai-chi ch'üan the *ch'i* permeates the bones and this is true T'ai-chi power.

Let ch'i circulate throughout the body freely and the body will be obedient to the mind.

Friends, if you desire your *ch'i* to circulate freely throughout your body, you must receive correct instruction in the Thirteen Postures. This is the art handed down by my late teacher. When executing the postures, the upper and lower body must relate naturally. If power is not forced, then and only then can the *ch'i* circulate freely. If the postures are natural, then the mind commands and the hands and feet follow.

If one can raise the spirit, there need be no fear of sluggishness or heaviness. This is what is meant by holding the head as if suspended from above.

The spirit is the master of the whole body. Not only in the martial arts, but in all pursuits, if the spirit is swift, one will never be sluggish or slow. Therefore, in speaking of the martial arts one must first mention raising the spirit. If we want to raise the spirit, then the head must be held erect with energy at the very crown. That is, the *ni-wan* point should be light and sensitive, with energy rising to the top. If you can awaken to this technique, you will understand what is meant by ''raising the spirit.''

Our feelings must become supremely sensitive in order for there to be complete and lively enjoyment. This is what is meant by the transformations of full and empty.

Feeling is that which circulates between the bones and the flesh. There is an indescribable kind of pleasure that comes from practicing the form and sparring. We must cause this circulating substance to fill the entire body, so that if we want it to go left it goes left, and if we want it to go right it goes right. This is what is meant by the changes of full and empty in T'ai-chi. The method of transforming the sense of feeling is like a half full bottle of water. If placed on its left side, the water rushes to the left; if placed on its right side, it rushes to the right. If this can be achieved, not only will you experience complete and lively enjoyment, but it will be as pleasurable as dance. When you have reached this stage, even if someone were to try to prevent you from practicing this art, they could not succeed. From this we can appreciate that the body receives infinite blessings.

When issuing energy one must sink, relax, be calm and concentrated in one direction.

When sparring with an opponent, first control his movement and then attack from one direction, the one in which he is losing his balance. When issuing energy, whether with the hand, shoulder or elbow, you must sink down, with the mind relaxed and calm. Issue energy by attacking the opponent in only one direction. If my energy is not scattered it will be easy to throw the opponent for a great distance.

Our posture should be erect and relaxed, able to control the eight directions.

When the head is erect and the *wei-lü* straight, the body will not incline. Our mental attitude should be relaxed and comfortable, with the idea of waiting for movement with stillness. The waist and legs are like a standing wheel and the shoulders and hands like a horizontal wheel. When they are able to rotate in circles at our will, then we will have control of the eight directions.

Directing the ch'i is like threading a pearl with nine bends in the hole. There is nowhere it does not penetrate.

The "nine-bends-pearl" is a pearl with a winding path within it. If we compare the human body to a pearl, it can be seen that the four limbs and hundred bones are all full of bends. If we can direct the *ch'i* into the limbs without any gaps, then the skill of threading the nine-bends-pearl will be ours.

*When energy is set in motion it is like steel
tempered a hundred times. What resistance will it
fail to defeat?*

Energy set in motion "like steel tempered a hundred times" is internal energy. It is not a skill acquired in one day. After days and months, little by little, it is gradually refined like a piece of crude iron which is tempered every day with pounding. Slowly it is transformed into pure steel. If a broadsword or two-edged sword is made from such steel, it will be incomparably sharp, and there is no "resistance it cannot defeat." The energy which T'ai-chi develops is both fine and strong and can destroy even an iron man. Of what concern, then, are opponents made of mere flesh and blood?

*You should appear like a falcon seizing a hare,
with the spirit of a cat catching a rat.*

The falcon is an animal capable of flight, a bird of prey. In the winter it is used for hunting. This passage means that in sparring with an opponent we should imitate the appearance of a bird of prey. When we spy our victim, our eyes should look as if we would immobilize it with our beak, and as soon as our hands make contact, we would control it in our clutches, just like a falcon catching its prey. This comparison is not meant to be abusive, but these are the words of my late teacher. Perhaps some explanation is in order. I hope that my readers will not be confused. When stalking rats, cats look just like tigers. They lie in wait, crouching with the weight on their rear legs. The vital spirit of their whole being is focused on the rat hole. When the rat emerges they pounce ferociously and capture him. This describes the posture in T'ai-chi which involves sinking the chest and raising the back, just like the cat stalking the rat. Wait for the chance, spring, and the opponent will be yours.

In stillness be like a great mountain; in movement like a mighty river.

After one has trained for a long time, the legs develop root and one's stance is like a mountain. Human force cannot shake us. The metaphor of the river expresses the infinite possibilities for transformation. One technique becomes five and five become a hundred. The flow is unceasing like a river.

Store energy like drawing a bow; release it like shooting an arrow.

To store energy means to reserve it. T'ai-chi energy is not external but stored internally. When squaring off with an opponent our internal energy has the fullness of a drawn bow or a ball filled with air. If the opponent touches my arm, although it feels soft as cotton, he cannot push it down. This greatly astonishes him. In the midst of his perplexity he is unaware that my bow already has a drawn arrow which is about to fly. At this moment I am like the bow, and my opponent becomes like the arrow. The energy is released so fast that the opponent is thrown with the speed of an arrow.

Seek the straight in the curved; store first and then issue. Power issues from the back; our steps must follow the body. To withdraw is to attack and to attack is to withdraw. After withdrawing reconnect again.

Allow me to summarize these lines with a simple explanation. "Seeking the straight in the curved" means that bending is followed by extension. "Store first and then issue," "Power issues from the back," and "To withdraw is to attack" are all based on a single principle. That is, our spirit should be like a cat stalking a rat. Students should be able to grasp this with a word or two.

*In moving to and fro use "fold up;" in advancing
and retreating use turns and changes.*

When sparring with an opponent, you should
sometimes move in and sometimes out. "Fold up"
refers to postures where the elbows are bent and the
forearms curved. Folding up turns the backside to the
opponent's body or hands. This technique is only useful
when in close with an opponent and useless at a
distance. In advancing and retreating do not get stuck in
a rut with just one posture, but turn and change
according to the situation.

*From the greatest softness comes the greatest
hardness. From the proper breathing comes
sensitivity and liveliness.*

We must use soft methods in practicing the Thirteen
Postures. When our art is perfected we will develop
internal energy, stored and concealed within this
softness. As for breathing, our inhalation has the ability
to lift a man up and cause an opponent's rear leg to leave
the ground. Again, with our exhalation, the power of
our *ch'i* traveling up the spine issues forth all the energy
of the entire body and can repel a man for a great
distance. When our breathing reaches this level of
perfection, then our physical movements become
sensitive, lively and fluid.

*The ch'i should be properly cultivated and not
damaged. Energy should be stored by rounding
and there will always be a surplus.*

Practicing T'ai-chi is actually a method for cultivating
ch'i and not the work of circulating *ch'i.* What is the
purpose of learning to circulate *ch'i*? With training
methods which involve stress, strength and anger, the
ch'i is concentrated in one place and it is not easy to
project. It is likely that there will be internal blocks. What

is the purpose of "cultivating *ch'i?*" Mencius said, "I excel at cultivating my great *ch'i.*" If you can eliminate haste and anxiety, this intrinsic *ch'i* will develop. Still the mind and nourish your original nature. When practicing, cause the inner sexual energy, *ch'i* and spirit to unite. Direct the *ch'i* to circulate through the "nine-bends-pearl." Even if one has not yet reaped the full benefits, it is certain that at least there will be no harm.

When sparring with opponents, never allow the forearm to be extended straight. If you can coordinate the upper and lower parts of the body, step with the changes of position, keep the arms rounded and maintain a surplus of power, then the opponent will quickly be thrown. This is what is meant by, "Energy should be stored by rounding and there will always be a surplus."

The mind is the commander, the ch'i a flag and the waist a banner.

T'ai-chi principles are like those for mobilizing troops in time of war. It is necessary to have commanders and flags to direct operations. It is the same with T'ai-chi: thus the mind is the commander, meaning that the mind directs the *ch'i.* If we can employ the *ch'i* like a flag, then whatever we will, the *ch'i* follows. The waist acting like a "banner" refers to the great banners carried by military troops. The small flags control movement and the great flags stillness. In martial arts methods the waist operates like the axle of a wheel and should not throw over or rend the great banner.

First seek expansion and later contraction; then you will arrive at impeccable technique.

Expansion means largeness and relaxation of the sinews and muscles. When first learning the form, seek to make your postures open and large. This serves to relax the sinews and invigorate the blood and facilitates building strength. After your strength is sufficient then begin to develop the external ability to unify the sinews, bones and muscles.

Internal concentration of the sexual energy, *ch'i* and spirit is what is meant by contraction. When both the inner and outer are developed together with transformations of movement and stillness, then you can proceed from expansion to contraction. If the body is strong and the understanding of applications complete, you can reach the level of impeccability. To speak of "large techniques" or "small techniques" is erroneous.

It is also said that things are first in the mind and later in the body.

When first learning to spar with an opponent, even if you concentrate your mind, probably you will not be successful. After you have perfected the art, then you can function without mental concentration. Wherever your body is attacked, you will be able to respond automatically. Without your even being consciously aware of what you are doing, the opponent will be thrown. At this level your hands and feet will move of themselves. At the outset of study it is in the mind, but after you have mastered the art, it is in the body. This is like when one is beginning to learn to calculate with an abacus. The mind first recites the mnemonic verse while the hands manipulate the beads. Later, when one is thoroughly familiar, the verse may be forgotten and the hand simply moves in response to the will. This is an example of being first in the mind and then in the hands. Martial arts principles are precisely the same.

The body should be relaxed and the ch'i will permeate the bones. The spirit should be open and the body calm.

Although you use concentration to relax the belly, strictly avoid rousing the energy. When the *ch'i* is trained, it will permeate the bones. The bones and muscles should be sunk and heavy. We should be like cotton on the outside and like bands of steel on the inside, or like iron concealed in cotton.

At all times bear in mind and consciously remember that as soon as one part of the body moves the whole body moves; and as soon as one part is still the whole body is still.

Never forget for a moment that as soon as one part of the body moves the whole body moves. Do not move just one part independently. This is like a train: when the engine moves, all of the cars follow. The movement of energy in T'ai-chi must be precisely coordinated. Although it is precisely coordinated, it must still be natural and lively, just like the moving cars in a train. Although the body is in motion, the mind should guard its stillness; and when the mind is still the whole body will be still. Although it is still, it also contains the potential for movement. The most important thing is that with every movement the upper and lower parts of the body move together.

Pushing and pulling, back and forth, the ch'i adheres to the back and permeates the spine. Inwardly strengthen your vital spirit and outwardly give the appearance of calm and ease.

''Pushing and pulling, back and forth'' refers to the dance-like movement of the hands. When you inhale, the *ch'i* adheres to the spine where it gathers waiting to be projected. This storing of *ch'i* in the spine is what is meant by ''inwardly strengthen your vital spirit.'' Your outward appearance is cultured, calm and at ease. Although you practice the martial arts you are still civil.

Step like a cat; move the energy like reeling silk from a cocoon.

In T'ai-chi ch'üan, our steps are as light and subtle as a cat's. When practicing our form, we move the energy as smoothly and continuously as reeling silk from a cocoon.

The attention of your whole being should be on the spirit and not on the ch'i. If it is on the ch'i, there will be blocks. Those whose attention is on the ch'i have no power; those whose attention is not on the ch'i achieve essential hardness.

The human body has three treasures. These are sexual energy (*ching*), *ch'i,* and spirit (*shen*). In T'ai-chi the attention is on the last of these. "Attention not being on the *ch'i* means it is not on the circulating *ch'i.* "If it is on the *ch'i* , there will be blocks" means that when circulating the *ch'i,* if it swells up in one place, then it will be blocked and insensitive. To say that, "Those whose attention is on the *ch'i* have no power" means that their *ch'i* is dead. I may feel that I have power, but my opponent knows that I have none. To say that "Those whose attention is not on the *ch'i* achieve essential hardness" means that without dead *ch'i* they possess soft strength. Wherever you direct the mind, power arrives. When you make contact with an opponent it is like thongs strapped to his arm. Thus without using strength, the opponent feels that our hands are as heavy as Mount T'ai. By not using direct power, marvelous power manifests. Those without dead *ch'i* achieve essential hardness.

Ch'i is like a wheel and the waist like an axletree.

The feeling of the whole body is like a moving wheel. The waist is the ruler of the whole body and rotates like an axletree. So all of the movements of our art are controlled by the waist.

It is also said that if the opponent does not move, you do not move. When the opponent makes the slightest move, you move first.

When sparring with an opponent, do not move, but wait for the opponent to move, and then move first.

Your energy seems relaxed but is not relaxed, about to expand but not yet expanded. Even when energy is released, mental continuity is maintained.

When one extends a hand to attack in T'ai-chi, we say it is relaxed, but it is not relaxed. In extending the limbs, never completely straighten them. When practicing the form, the idea of continuity applies to prescribed postures which are threaded together in a series. However, if we are talking about sparring and practical applications, there are no prescribed postures for repelling an opponent. Externally my posture may appear to have an end point but my consciousness never slacks for a moment.

When you break a lotus root in half, the fine strands of fiber do not break. This comparison should make my meaning clear. Master Yang often said, ''The energy is released, but the mental continuity is maintained; the lotus root is broken, but the fibers are intact.''

The Method of Achieving
Perfect Clarity in T'ai-chi

Using energy is not correct;
Not using strength is not correct.
To be soft but hard is correct.

Leaning away is not correct;
Butting in is not correct.
Not leaning away and not butting in
    is correct.

Sticking is not correct;
Not sticking is not correct.
Being neither over-anxious
    nor separating is correct.

Floating is not correct;
Heaviness in not correct.
Lightness, sensitivity, relaxation
    and sinking are correct.

Bravery is not correct;
Timidity is not correct.
Strong courage and keen perception
    are correct.

Striking people is not correct;
Not striking people is not correct.
Causing the opponent to mentally
    surrender is correct.

Wang Tsung-yüeh's
Treatise on T'ai-chi ch'üan

Note: Pay attention to practice. The
commentary is not just writing
for the sake of writing.

*T'ai-chi [The Great Ultimate] is born of Wu-chi
[The Infinite] and is the mother of yin and yang.*

Non-action is Wu-chi; action is T'ai-chi. When the *ch'i* stirs in the void, T'ai-chi is born and divides into *yin* and *yang* . Therefore, in practicing T'ai-chi we must first discuss *yin* and *yang*, for they embrace all phenomena. From mutual production and mutual destruction comes change. T'ai-chi is born of Wu-chi and is the mother of *yin* and *yang*.

*In motion they separate; in stillness
they become one.*

When we practice T'ai-chi, as soon as the will moves, it is projected into the four limbs. T'ai-chi gives birth to *yin* and *yang*, the four duograms, eight trigrams and the Palace of Nine. This is equivalent to Ward-off, Roll-back, Press, Push, Pull-down, Split, Elbow-stroke, Shoulder-stroke, Advance, Retreat, Gaze-left, Look-right and Central Equilibrium. When we are still, all reverts to Wu-chi; the mind and spirit unite as one. The whole body is completely empty and we become aware of the slightest touch.

*Avoid both excess and insufficiency; extend when
the opponent bends and bend when he extends.*

Whether practicing the form or sparring, avoiding excess and insufficiency is equally applicable. Excess means going too far and insufficiency means not going far enough. Excess and insufficiency are both departures from the center. If the opponent attacks, give way by bending. Bending means to arch. If the opponent has not yet gone on the attack and attempts to retreat, then I follow him and extend. Extending means to issue energy with the hands. Excess can be seen in the error of butting and insufficiency in losing contact. The inability to bend is belligerence; the inability to extend is separation. Conscientiously remember the four words: losing contact, butting, belligerence and separation. If your art can be free of over-anxiousness and separation, you will be able to perform marvels with your hands.

The opponent is hard while I am soft. This is yielding. I am yielding while the opponent is resistant. This is adhering.

For example, if two people are sparring and the other person is hard and direct, then I use soft hands to cover the opponent's. I firmly cover his energy, like a beating whip. It will be extremely difficult for him to throw me off. My contact is like a rubber band which binds up his ability to release or expand. If he uses great force, I stick to his wrist and shift my weight to the rear. At the same time, without separating, I receive the incoming force and turn the waist a half circle to neutralize it. I extend my hand towards his left side, causing it to be power-less. I am yielding while he is resistant. By adhering to the opponent I prevent him from escaping.

There is an old story that tells of a wild monk who excelled at using head butts. He was about to try conclusions with a man who knew his reputaion as an invincible ram-butter and was extremely intimidated. Now this man noticed that the monk had freshly shaven his head and suddenly thought of a plan. He went into the house and got a wet washcloth. When the monk attempted his butting technique, the man tossed the washcloth over his head, and pulling down, he threw the monk for a fall. This is the principle of the soft overcoming the hard.

Respond to speed with speed and slowness with slowness.

At present most of my fellow T'ai-chi practitioners understand the art of yielding but do not understand the method of quick response. I am afraid they would fare badly against external stylists. ''Speed'' means quickness; ''slowness'' means to be deliberate. If the opponent approaches slowly, I respond with yielding and following. This principle is very clear. If the opponent comes at me with great speed, how can I use yielding? In this case, I must respond by using the method of T'ai-chi ''intercept energy'' and the principle of ''not late and not early.'' It is just like concealing troops in ambush to intercept the enemy. What do we mean by ''not late and not early?'' When the opponent has already launched his attack, but has not yet landed, I intercept his arm with my hand before it becomes straight. This will immediately deflect the attack. This is how to repulse a frontal attack. Without receiving the true transmission, ''responding to speed with speed'' is impossible.

Although the changes are infinite, the principles remain the same.

When sparring with opponents, whether push-hands or free-hand, no matter how we reckon it, the principles are: the great circle, the small circle, the half circle, the marvel of *yin* and *yang*, full and empty in the feet, the T'ai-chi *yin-yang* fishes, and maintaining vertical. Though we flow unceasingly through myriad changes, the priciples of T'ai-chi remain the same.

*From mastery of the postures, you will gradually
awaken to interpreting energy. From interpreting
energy, you will arrive at spiritual insight.
However, without long arduous practice, you will
not suddenly make this breakthrough.*

"Postures" refers to the T'ai-chi form. At present my
fellow practitioners seek only to grasp interpreting
energy, but are unable to repulse opponents. Instead,
they should first learn the postures correctly and
practice them until thoroughly mastered. Then
gradually they should study interpreting energy. The
ancients had a saying that to ignore the root and trim
the branches was like raising a square inch of wood
above the highest building. This teaches us that we
must first develop the postures and later learn
interpreting energy. It will then not be difficult to
reach "spiritual insight." Spiritual insight here refers to
miraculous martial skill; "sudden breakthrough"
means grasping the marvelous secrets of martial art. If
you can circulate the *ch'i* through the "nine-bends-
pearl," then you will have mastered the principles of
T'ai-chi. Without long practice and familiarity, how can
you hope to reach this level?

*There is a light and sensitive energy at the crown
of the head; sink the ch'i to the tan-t'ien; do not
lean or incline.*

The "crown of the head" refers to the very top.
Taoists call this point the *ni-wan* ["clay pill"], or what is
generally called the *t'ien-men* ["heavenly gate"]. It
should feel empty and the head should be held erect.
The spirit rises, but do not let the *ch'i* reach the crown.
After long practice, the eyes will be bright and one will
never suffer headaches. The *tan-t'ien* is located a little
more than an inch below the navel in the belly. This is
where all the intrinsic *ch'i* in the body gathers. When we

120

move, it issues from this source as from a sea of *ch'i* and circulates throughout the four limbs. When *ch'i* is made to revert to the *tan-t'ien*, the body and *ch'i* do not "lean or incline." Leaning and inclining is like a porcelain jar full of water. If the jar is upset, the water will spill out. If the *tan-t'ien* leans or inclines, then the *ch'i* cannot revert and gather. The Buddhists call this method "holy relics" [*she-li-tzu*, the gem-like remains after cremation of one who has achieved Buddhahood] and Taoists call it "cultivating the elixir" (*lien-tan*).

Practicing in this way, one will become strong and virile. After long effort, the sinews and bones will appear soft on the outside with strength and substance concealed within. When the *ch'i* is strong, one is impervious to the hundred ailments.

Suddenly disappear and suddenly appear. If the opponent puts pressure on the left, become empty on the left; if he puts pressure on the right, become empty on the right.

"Disappearing" means to conceal; "appearing" means to expose. The method of disappearing and appearing in sparring is most subtle and difficult to fathom. When an opponent attempts to attack me, I withdraw and "suddenly disappear," which prevents him from being able to apply his force. Now when he pulls his hand back, I follow him and advance, suddenly appearing. The opponent has no idea if my posture will be high or low, or whether I will attack from above or below. He will be helpless to withstand my thrust.

Practicing T'ai-chi is like a small boat on a river. When a man steps into it, it leans to one side and seems to suddenly disappear, but when the man is aboard, it rises again, suddenly reappearing. It is also like the transformations of the dragon which mounts on high and then descends. When it comes down, it disappears by concealing itself in physical forms. Then it again reappears, soaring into the heavens, riding the clouds and revealing itself. This principle expresses the idea that T'ai-chi can rise and it can fall. "Disappearing and appearing" is the theory of suddenly existing and suddenly not existing.

Those who are heavy cannot move. Is it possible not to move when sparring with opponents? To engage in martial arts, we must have active bodies. Our hands and feet must be nimble; only then can we meet an adversary. If the opponent attacks my left side, I incline slightly, become empty and give him nothing to take advantage of. If he attacks my right side, I withdraw my right shoulder, giving his fist nothing to land on. My body is nimble and impossible to catch. This is the idea of becoming empty on the left, if the left is attacked; and vanishing on the right, if the right is attacked.

*Looking upward, it seems higher and higher;
looking downward, it seems deeper and deeper.
Advancing, it seems further and further;
retreating, it seems shorter and shorter.*

"Looking upward" means high and "looking downward" means low. If the opponent seeks to attack from a high position, I become so tall he cannot reach me; if the opponent seeks to push me down, I descend so low that he loses his center of gravity. Saying to yourself, "looking upward it seems higher and higher," look up with your eyes and imagine throwing the opponent on top of the building. Saying, "looking downward, it seems deeper and deeper," imagine beating the opponent into the earth.

There is a story concerning Master Yang Pan-hou. On a summer day he was in a field outside a small village (a granary in north China) cooling himself. All of a sudden a man appeared, saluted, and asked the whereabouts of Pan-hou. He replied that he was the same, when without warning the man attacked him violently with three fingers. Pan-hou noticed that there was a grass hut in the field about seven feet high, so he motioned with his hand saying, "Friend, why don't you go up there?" With that, he threw him on top of the hut. Then he said, "Please come down, go home and find medical treatment." A villager asked him how he was able to throw the man on top of the hut. He responded, "Looking up it is higher and higher," but the villager could not comprehend his meaning.

In north China there was a man named Lo Wan-tzu who was a student of Pan-hou. After studying for a number of years, he wanted to test his art. Master Pan-hou asked him how he would like to be thrown into the shape of a silver ingot, like those of the Yüan dynasty. Wan laughed and invited him to try. They engaged, and he ended up, just as Pan-hou had said, with both hands and feet pointing towards the sky and the right side of his hip facing down, precisely in the shape of a Yüan ingot. Although he was not literally thrown under the earth, he did suffer a hip dislocation. He was cured, but to this day he still has a bit of a limp. This man is a fine martial artist and is alive today. He often says, "Look down and it is deeper and deeper" is indeed a fearful technique.

A feather cannot be added to the body nor a fly alight.

After training for a long time you feel so sensitive and alert that you become aware of the slightest touch. You cannot bear the touch of even something as light as a feather. Even a tiny fly cannot alight on my body, for it would be like landing on the inside of a finely glazed jar which was so slippery that the fly could not stand. I use my neutralizing power to make the fly's legs skid out from under it. This can truly be called the culmination of skill in T'ai-chi.

There is a story that tells how Pan-hou used to lie under the shade of a tree to rest during the summer when he was training. Once a wind came up and blew some leaves down, but not one of them could alight on his body and they slid off to the ground. He used to test his skill by opening his shirt and lying down on his bed. Then he would take a pinch of millet and place it on his navel. We would hear an exhaling sound and the grains would shoot out like pellets from a crossbow striking the ceiling of the tiled roof. Pan-hou's art was truly supreme. My friends, strive earnestly to match it.

My opponent does not know me, but I know him. Wherever the hero goes, he is unmatched. This is the goal to which we aspire.

When sparring with opponents, we do not use prescribed postures, but make it impossible for them to lay a hand on us. We use the great general, Chu Ke-liang's, military strategy of alternating offense and defense, so that the enemy cannot predict our movements. There is a proverb that goes, "They cannot guess what kind of medicine I am selling from my gourd." The opponent does not know that I have mastered T'ai-chi's technique of sizing up an opponent. If one is very familiar with interpreting energy, then the hand becomes miraculously sensitive. When the opponent makes the slightest movement, I anticipate it, and following his hand employ deft skill to attack and repel him. If we have not yet closed, I use the method of sizing up the opponent and visually ascertain his movement. Sun Tzu's *Art of War (Sun Tzu ping-fa)* states: "Know yourself and know the enemy; a hundred battles, a hundred victories." "Wherever the hero goes he is unmatched. This is the goal to which we aspire."

*There are many other schools of martial arts.
Although there are differences in style, they do
not go beyond strength bullying weakness and
slowness giving way to speed, the strong beating
the weak and slow hands yielding to fast. All
of this is native physical endowment and has
nothing to do with what is acquired through
serious study.*

Although there are numerous schools in the martial arts, and each has its own postures and applications, to sum up, what they all have in common is an emphasis on speed and strength. In this way, they are simply working with inherited ability and not the results of study. There are many famous men in the various schools, but they cannot approach the subtlety and marvelousness of T'ai-chi's principles.

*If we examine the concept of four ounces repelling
a thousand pounds, it is clear that it is not brute
force that prevails.*

The sages have taught us that to conquer with force leaves the heart unconquered. When we learn the art of weakness overcoming strength, of slowness overcoming speed, and using skill to control an opponent, then we truly conquer the opponent's heart. Moreover, we will have no regrets for our arduous study. Practicing T'ai-chi ch'üan enables us to attract the opponent while giving his brute force nothing to land on. Even a thousand pounds of force is useless. Only when we are sensitive and lively can we demonstrate the marvel of giving an opponent nothing to land on. When we are able to attract an opponent and give his force nothing to land on, then we will possess the marvel of four ounces repelling a thousand pounds.

Many years ago there was a story about a wealthy old man who lived west of Peking and whose estate was as big as a city. People called it "Chang's little prefecture." Chang loved the martial arts and kept more than thirty boxers as bodyguards in his house. He himself by nature was also eager to study. He heard that there was a famous man in Kuang-p'ing Prefecture named Yang Lu-ch'an and begged a friend, Wu Lu-ch'ing, to go to him and extend an invitation. When Yang arrived, Chang noticed he was very thin and barely five feet tall. His appearance was honest and generous and his clothes were very plain. Chang greeted him with little ceremony and the banquet in his honor was far from sumptuous. Master Yang understood all this and ate and drank by himself without paying attention to anything. Chang was very displeased and said, "I have often heard my boxers mention your great name. Can T'ai-chi really be used to defeat an opponent? Lu-ch'an knew that modesty would not do, so he said, "There are three kinds of men who cannot be beaten." Chang asked what he meant by these three kinds, and Yang replied, "Those cast of bronze, those pounded of iron, and those made of wood. These three are difficult to beat, but everyone else is no problem." Chang said, "I have thirty men in my keep and Master Liu is first among them. He is so strong he can lift five hundred pounds. Would you like to play with him?" Yang said there would be no harm in trying. Liu came at him with the fury of Mount T'ai and his fists made a whizzing sound. As he approached, Yang used his right hand to neutralize and his left to pat him. The man was thrown for three yards. Chang rubbed his fist and said, "You, Sir, are possessed of a miraculous art." With that he ordered his cooks to start fresh and prepare a full banquet of Manchu and Chinese dishes. He respected him from that point as his own teacher. Liu was as strong as a bull, but without skill, how could he compete? From this we can see the results of applying "clearly it is not force that prevails."

When we see an old man successfully defending himself against a large number of men, what has this to do with speed?

An "old man" may be considered one in his seventies or eighties. Being able to "successfully defend himself against a large number of men" indicates that he has practiced T'ai-chi ch'üan. Without practicing it is difficult for even a man in his prime to defeat one or two men. If one continues to practice from the very first day of study until old age, one's sinews and bones will remain strong and the *ch'i* and blood full and abundant. Thus a man of seventy or eighty can defeat a whole crowd. Like old General Huang Chung, who at the battle of Ting-chün Mountain said, "The man may be old but the horse is not; the horse may be old but the sword is not." His words are very strong. Those who practice T'ai-chi ch'üan may become old in years but their spirit is young and they can defeat many men. This is the basic idea.

There is an old story about Master Yang Chien-hou. One day right after a rain storm there was a narrow path just wide enough for one person to get through all the mud in the courtyard. A student named Chao was standing on the path looking up at the sky without realizing that the old Master had come out of the house and was walking up behind him. Chien-hou wanted to play a joke, so he put out his right hand and lightly pressed on Chao's right shoulder. Chao felt as if a great roofbeam had been lowered on him and his body collapsed to the side of the path. The old Master laughed but said nothing and went on his way.

Another day Chien-hou was standing in the courtyard speaking to a group of students when he decided to have some fun with them. Some eight or nine students were pressing around him when the old Master turned his body a few times and the whole crowd was thrown helter skelter, some for more than ten feet and some for eight or nine. The old man was close to eighty at the time. So to say that "an old man can successfully defend himself against a large number" is not hyperbole. The word "speed" in the sentence, "What has this to do with speed" refers to chaotic speed which is simply wild and confused. Wild and confused speed is useless. To be without speed is not good, but speed only becomes useful with skill.

Stand like a sensitive balance; move actively like a wheel.

To "stand like a sensitive balance" means to stand erect and without leaning. Only then can you control the eight directions, which correspond to the eight trigrams of the *I ching*, or the four sides and four corners of the square. To "move actively like a wheel" refers to the continuous circulation of the *ch'i*. The ancients said, "Find the center of the circle and you can respond to any situation." The waist is like an axletree and the four limbs like a wheel. If the waist cannot act like an axletree then the limbs cannot revolve around it. If you want to make the axle rotate, it should be well lubricated. Colleagues who carefully consider this will grasp it for themselves. There is no need to belabor it.

If you keep your weight on one side you will be able to follow; if you are double-weighted you will be clumsy.

In the commentary above, we used the metaphor of the wheel. If you use one foot to push down on a wheel it will naturally follow the wheel around. Double-weightedness would be like using the right foot to press on the right side and the left leg on the left side. If the two pressures are equal, naturally it will be blocked and unable to rotate. This principle is very obvious and requires no further elaboration.

We often see people who have faithfully studied this art for several years but cannot neutralize an attack and most often are bested by an opponent. This is simply because they have not yet corrected the error of double-weighting.

Friends, you can gain a great deal from a very simple explanation. Let us consider, for example, a few people who have practiced T'ai-chi every day for five or six years, but who are always bested in competition. A colleague asked, "You have studied faithfully for five or six years, but why are you still not successful? Please demonstrate the Thirteen Postures so I can see." What we see in his form is "horse stances," clenched fists, a fierce countenance, and gritted teeth. He has as much strength as an ox but his *ch'i* is nowhere to be seen. This is the result of practicing double-weighted. A colleague laughed and said, "You, Sir, have simply failed to understand the error of double-weightedness." Another man said, "I have been practicing without using force for five or six years, but why is it that I cannot even knock over a ten year old kid?" The colleague asked him to demonstrate the Thirteen Postures and noticed that indeed he used no force at all. However, he was floating like goose down and didn't dare to extend his hands or feet. He was even afraid to open his eyes wide. The colleague laughed and said, "You, Sir, are guilty of the error of 'double-floating.' Double-weightedness is an error and double-floating is also an error." Everyone laughed and asked, "How can we discover the true method of practice?"

You must seek to avoid this error.

The errors of double-weightedness and double-floating must be avoided. Now this is quite easy to accomplish. With this manual, it is not difficult to understand. First read the training methods in this book through once. The principles are many and cannot be comprehended in one reading. From then on you can practice for ten days and read this book for one. Little by little the benefits of this book will make themselves known. If you have difficulty understanding any passage you can ask a qualified teacher.

You must know yin and yang. To adhere is to yield; to yield is to adhere. Yin never leaves yang and yang never leaves yin. When yin and yang complement each other, this is interpreting energy.

Yin and *yang* are empty and full. To summarize, adhere, connect, yield to neutralize and interpret the opponent's incoming energy. This has been thoroughly explained above and need not be repeated.

After learning to interpret energy, the more you practice the more your skill advances. Silently memorize and thoroughly ponder. Little by little you will reach the stage where the body will automatically follow the mind.

The ability to interpret an opponent's incoming energy plus daily practice refer to the process of training and mastery over a long period. To "thoroughly ponder" means to seek insight into the practical applications taught by the teacher. When these have become completely familiar, simply put out the hands and whatever the mind conceives will be accomplished. Then you will have reached the stage of the body automatically following the mind.

The root of all is to give up yourself and follow others.

When sparring with opponents, you know that you must follow the other person's movements and not move independently. My teacher, Yang Ch'eng-fu often said that to move on one's own was clumsy, but to follow another was nimble. If you can follow another, you can acquire the marvelous ability to neutralize energy. If you follow others, you cannot go off independently. Only when you are able to follow others can you be independent. This principle is extremely real and extremely subtle.

Most people make the mistake of scorning what is near and pursuing what is far. The slightest error will take you a thousand miles off course. Students must finely discriminate; hence the reason for this treatise.

In sparring with opponents, most people neglect what is near in favor of what is distant. Using stillness to wait for movement and striking when the opportunity arises is based on the idea of the near. Moving up and down looking for a place to attack is based on the idea of the far. Skill in T'ai-chi is a matter of inches at the most and millimeters at the least. Therefore there is no room for error. An error of one millimeter is like missing the mark by a thousand miles. Fellow T'ai-chi players must pay special attention to this.

The above are the teachings on T'ai-chi ch'üan transmitted by Wang Tsung-yüeh.

A Critical Note

Some people claim that teachers, whether academic or martial, always hold something back in transmitting their knowledge. I am of a different opinion. Both in the academic field and the martial arts, regardless if one is teaching friends or students, there are two things to consider. A longtime friend will develop great respect and a student will remember his master for a hundred years. So it would be completely unnatural for a teacher not to give his utmost to his students. It is just that students of the martial arts tend to be self-righteous and often abandon their studies in mid-course. To say then that the teacher is unwilling to share his secrets or is holding something back is a very peculiar theory. In reality, the essence of T'ai-chi is not found in the external postures, but rather in the internal principles, energy and *ch'i*. Only when one has grasped the principles and thoroughly apprehended and assimilated them can one's art be complete.

The Eight Gates and Five Steps

Positions	*Eight Gates*
Ward-off (south)	K'an
Roll-back (west)	Li
Press (east)	Tui
Push (north)	Chen
Pull-down (northwest)	Hsün
Split (southeast)	Ch'ien
Elbow-stroke (northeast)	K'un
Shoulder-stroke (southwest)	Ken

The positions and gates represent the principle of *yin* and *yang* reversing positions. They move around and around in continuous cycle. It is indispensable to understand the four sides of the square and four corners. Ward-off, Roll-back, Press and Push are the four side techniques; Pull-down, Split, Elbow-stroke and Shoulder-stroke are the four corner techniques. Combining the corner and side techniques, we get the trigrams of the gates and positions. The steps correspond to the Five Elements and give us control of the eight directions. The Five Elements are Advance (fire), Retreat (water), Gaze-left (wood), Look-right (metal) and Central Equilibrium (earth). Advance and Retreat belong to fire; Gaze-left and Look-right belong to wood and metal. Central Equilibrium acts as the pivot point. It contains the eight trigrams for the feet and the Five Elements for the hands and steps. The number is eight plus five. Thirteen derives from nature. Hence the Thirteen Postures are called the Eight Gates and Five Steps.

How To Work on the
Eight Gates and Five Steps

The eight trigrams and Five Elements are a part of man's natural endowment. We must first understand the basis of work: conscious movement. Only after grasping conscious movement are we able to interpret energy, and only after interpreting energy can we reach the level of spiritual insight. Thus the first stage of our work is understanding conscious movement, which although it is a natural endowment is extremely difficult for us to acquire.

The Above and Below in T'ai-chi
May be Called Heaven and Earth

The "four techniques," above and below,
  divide into Heaven and earth.
Pull-down, Split, Elbow-stroke and Shoulder-
  stroke each have their origin and object.
Pull-down being Heaven and Shoulder-stroke
  earth, they mutually respond to each other.
Why should we care if above and below
  do not complement each other?
If Split and Elbow-stroke are practiced
  too far apart,
One will lose the relation of *Ch'ien* [Heaven],
  and *K'un* [earth] and will lament it forever.
This theory explains the planes of
  Heaven and earth.
When advancing use Elbow-stroke and Split,
  with the arms in the shape of the character
  for man [i.e., bent].

Explanation of Eight, Five,
the Thirteen Postures and Long Boxing

In the training process, after one masters the individual postures, they should be connected in a flowing and continuous series. This is why it is called Long Boxing. However, if one does not acquire the ability to direct energy, there is the possibility of falling into a "slippery style" or perhaps a "hard style." Therefore, absolutely maintain softness, unity of the whole body and spirit, mind and *ch'i* as the root. After a long time you will naturally achieve mastery and reach any goal you set out for. What resistance can stand up to us?

When sparring with opponents, there are four words of primary importance, and these derive from the Eight Gates and Five Steps. With four standing hand techniques, the hands move like rolling millstones. Then there are the four techniques for Advance and Retreat, for Central Equilibrium, for high and low, for the techniques of Heaven, earth and man which rise from bottom to top, and the four techniques of Long Boxing. Begin with large and open postures and work up to small compact postures. When your extensions and contractions are completely free, then you will reach the intermediate and advanced levels of skill. Although soft, you will possess strength.

An Explanation of the Reversal of *Yin* and *Yang* in T'ai-chi

Yang is the trigram *Ch'ien,* Heaven, the sun, fire, the trigram *Li,* releasing, going out, issuing, facing, opening, a subordinate, flesh, application, materiality, the body, and martial arts. (All of the above has to do with establishing life). *Yin* is the trigram *K'un,* earth, water, moon, the trigram *K'an,* curling, entering, gathering, waiting, combining, the ruler, bones, essence, principle, mind and civil pursuits. (All of the above has to do with fulfilling one's nature). Inhaling and retreating represent the principle of the reversal of *yin* and *yang.*

If we examine the two words, water and fire, we will understand more clearly. Fire's flames tend to rise while water seeks the lowest level. If, however, we put fire under water, then their positions have been reversed. However, if we do not use some method to regulate them, then there will be no success. Now, if, for example, we place the water in a pot and place this over the fire, then the water inside will be heated by the fire. Thus, not only will the water not sink down, but it will borrow warmth from the fire. At the same time, although the flames of the fire rise, being covered by the pot which sets a limit, it is prevented from burning out of control and the water is kept from continually seeping away. This is called the principle of water and fire complementing each other, or the principle of reversal.

If we allow the fire to rise and the water to sink, the two will separate. This is why we seek to put them into a complementary relationship. This, then, is the principle of separating into two and recombining into one. Therefore it is said, "from one to two and from two to one." Summarizing this principle is the concept of three: or Heaven, earth and man. If one can understand the principle of the reversal of *yin* and *yang*, then we can begin to discuss the *tao*. When one understands the *tao* and can maintain this without lapse, then we can begin to discuss man. When one can magnify the *tao* by means of man, and know that the *tao* is not apart from man, then we can begin to discuss the unity of Heaven and earth. Heaven is above and earth below; man occupies the center. If one can explore the Heavens and examine the earth, unite with the brightness of the sun and the moon, be one with the five sacred mountains, the four great rivers, prime and decline, and the alternation of the four seasons, participate in the flowering and the withering of the trees and grasses, fathom the fortunes of ghosts and gods, and understand the rise and fall of human events, then we can speak of *Ch'ien* and *K'un* as the macrocosmic Heaven and earth and man as the microcosmic Heaven and earth.

Extend your knowledge and investigate the world through the wisdom and abilities of Heaven and earth. This, then, may be called man's innate wisdom and skill. If one's thoughts never depart from the truth, they will have a powerful effect. If one's great *ch'i* is properly nourished and not damaged, it will endure forever. This is what we mean by the body of man comprising a Heaven and earth in miniature. Heaven is one's nature and earth one's life. The light and sensitive in man is his spirit. If the spirit is not pure, how can one fulfill the role of third partner along with Heaven and earth? What is the meaning of existence if one does not fulfill one's nature, cultivate life, expand the spirit, and evolve positively?

Sizing Up an Opponent

When squaring off with an opponent, first observe whether his physique is great or small. If it is great, then he must have considerable brute strength, and I should respond with superior skill. If he is of slight build, then he will be skillful, and I must attack with power. In this way, I overcome the weak with strength and the mighty with cleverness. Regardless of size, if my opponent adopts high postures, then I must make use of low postures; if he adopts low postures, then I make use of high ones. This is the method of high and low, *yin* and *yang*.

In observing an opponent's movements, I first take note of his eyes and secondly his body and hands. If an opponent seeks to strike with the fist, I first observe his shoulders or his drawback. If the opponent attempts a kick, his body will first incline, thus indicating his intentions. Seeing this in advance, how can I fail to prevail? If the opponent approaches with a friendly countenance, I neutralize him with softness, but if he springs at me with an angry look, this indicates his evil intentions and I use all my strength to strike him. In this way, I am simply returning in kind what he has given me. Practitioners of T'ai-chi ch'üan are courteous at first and only aggressive if pressed.

In sparring we find that opponents vary greatly accordingly to speed. If my opponent's hands are slow, I must stick, join, adhere and follow. If my opponent's hands are fast and he strikes wildly, then I must keep my mind calm, my courage strong, and observe his final blow as it approaches. Concentrating on one place, I neutralize to the left and right and return the strike. There is a saying that "only a sensitive hand can walk a goat on a tether." This is the principle in T'ai-chi ch'üan of responding to speed with speed and following slowness with slowness.

There is more than one method for sparring with opponents. If my opponent has not yet come within close range, I first make contact with the hands while advancing with the feet. I neutralize and stick, stick and neutralize. If the opponent is skillful in escaping, I dare not pursue him, but adopt one of the Thirteen Postures and wait. I do not chase him when he escapes, but am like a tiger lying in ambush for the deer. When an opponent's movements are irregular and unpredictable, I remain at the very center of the Great Ultimate. I emphasize stillness and stability while my opponent emphasizes movement and anxiousness. The fire of anxiousness flares up and knows no forebearance, but I attack with complete composure. This is an example of mutual production and destruction. I have no difficulty in penetrating my opponent's inner defense. Thus the Great Ultimate gives birth to *yin* and *yang*, the four duograms and eight trigrams. This is fixed and eternal.

Introduction to the History of the Transmission of the T'ai-chi Spear

The Immortal, Master Chang San-feng, was practicing the Taoist arts in the Wutang Mountains. When at rest he meditated, training his spirit and returning to the Original Source; when active he roamed among the Three Mountains and Five Peaks. Every morning the Immortal repaired to a secluded spot at the top of the mountain where he gleaned the finest elements and subtle *ch'i* of Heaven and earth and circulated them with breathing exercises.

One day the Immortal suddenly saw a burst of golden light where the clouds meet the mist shrouded peaks. A thousand rays of marvelous *ch'i* spun and danced in the

Great Void. The Immortal hurried to the spot but saw nothing. He searched where the golden light had touched down and found a mountain stream and cave. Approaching the mouth of the cave, two golden snakes with flashing eyes emerged. The Immortal swished his duster and the golden light came down. He gazed upon it and realized that it was two long spears about seven feet five inches. They seemed to be made of rattan, but were not rattan; seemed of wood, but were not of wood. Their quality was such that swords could not harm them and they could be soft or hard at will. A rare glow emanated from within, and looking deeper, he found a book. Its title was *T'ai-chi Stick-Adhere Spear* and its destiny was to be transmitted to the world. He grasped the principles in the book and analyzed all of its marvels. All of the words in the book were written in the form of poems and songs. Today we cannot understand all the principles and marvels of the spear, but Master Chang extracted the essence of every word and transformed them into a series of postures. All men can now study and learn this art.

An Exposition of the Martial, Civil and Three Levels of T'ai-chi

In speaking of the *tao*, there is nowhere to begin but from cultivation of the self. The method of self-cultivation may be divided into three teachings. Each teaching represents a level of attainment. The highest level is great attainment, the lowest level is small attainment and the middle level is that of sincerity. There are three levels of attainment, but the accomplishment is one.

The civil is cultivated internally and the martial externally. Physical culture is internal and martial arts are external. When one's cultivation of the internal and the external results in superior accomplishments, this is the highest level of attainment. If one attains martial art

139

through the civil aspect of physical culture or the civil aspect of physical culture through the martial arts, this is the middle level of attainment. The lowest level, then, is knowing physical culture without the martial aspect or practicing only martial arts without physical culture.

A Story of Master Yang Lu-ch'an

After Master Yang Lu-ch'an had received the secret transmission, his nature was tranquil and his character loyal and generous. When his family had a bit extra, he would give generously to friends. One day a certain friend asked to borrow a hundred dollars to help him get by, saying he would return it next year. Master Lu-ch'an deliberately joked with him saying, ''Since you're borrowing this money, can you do me a favor? Grab the end of my spear and I will catapult you to the rooftop. If you do not land squarely on your feet, the loan is void.'' The man agreed. Master Yang then used his mind to mobilize his *ch'i,* and with one fling, the man landed on the rooftop. He was dumbfounded and stood there like a wooden man with his body bent forward. The Master laughed and fetched a ladder. When the man came down, he said that he was truly amazed. The Master laughed and said that it was just a game and gave the man a hundred dollars. The man departed well pleased with the outcome.

A Story of Imperial Tutor Yang Ch'ien-hou

Some time ago in Sian there was a prominent official named Chi Ssu who was very fond of the martial arts and eager to study. He heard that Master Yang had received the secret transmission of Wutang, so he traveled to the capital and invited the Master to stay in his home. Within a little more than a month he was introduced to hand techniques and spear and sword applications. Master often discussed the principle of the

140

superiority of stillness and softness with him. As a result Master's fame spread further than ever.

In Shensi there was a man named Great Sword Wang whose nickname was Bravo of the Red Inn. He could lift five hundred pounds and cover three hundred miles in one day. He excelled at the broadsword and loved the great spear. He was the foremost martial artist in Shensi and had more than five hundred students. When he heard Chi speak of Master Yang, he was skeptical and went to challenge him to a contest. Master, however, declined saying, ''Master Wang, you have trained diligently for a long time. I am afraid I am not your equal.'' Wang took Master as a coward and pressed him saying, ''I have heard of T'ai-chi ch'üan for a long time, but I wonder if T'ai-chi spear can be put to practical use?''

Master felt he had no choice, so smiling he nodded his assent, fetched his spear and entered the courtyard. Wang lunged at Master's chest, but he turned his body and rolled back. Wang pinned his spear and began to apply pressure, but Master remained empty. When Wang drew back his spear and was going in for the kill, Master took advantage of his incoming energy and used the ''scooping'' technique to stun him. Without knowing what happened, Wang's spear went up as straight as an incense stick and he wounded himself in the face. He landed face up about six or seven paces away. Rising, he apologized saying, ''From now on I will respect your miraculous power.'' He completely abandoned his own methods and followed Master Yang. He studied for a long time very conscientiously. Having met his superior, he was able to study without jealousy, and was not ashamed to be humble though he had a great reputation himself.

MISCELLANEOUS COMMENTS

There was a man who wanted to study the martial arts and asked which were better, the internal or external schools. I answered that all of the systems handed down by the ancient masters were good, and it was simply a question of receiving a true transmission or not. He asked again saying, ''Which is better, the Wutang or Shaolin school?'' I answered that if he wanted to learn Wutang, then he should study T'ai chi, and if he wanted to study Shaolin, he should study Shaolin. Everyone should follow their own inclination.

There was a man who wanted to know how many years it took to learn T'ai-chi ch'üan. I said, ''My friend, when it comes to the martial arts, one cannot speak in terms of years. A teacher may use the same methods to transmit his knowledge, but each student's capacity is different. Some learn in a year or two; some master it in just three to five months. There are also those who fail to understand it after ten or twenty years. Excellence in this art is not a matter of physical stature or age, but exclusively the individual's intelligence. I have studied this art for fifteen years, but often feel the need to appeal to teachers.

The Secret of Martial Arts Study

Respect the art and respect the teacher,
And you will naturally receive the
   true transmission.
Slight the art and slight the teacher,
And you might as well not waste your time.

A Story of Yang Lu-ch'an

When Master Lu-ch'an was in the capital, there was a boxer adept at using pressure points, who heard of Master and wanted to challenge him. When he tested his skill, Master Lu-ch'an quickly caught his wrist and used the "sinew-seizing" technique. The opponent was unable to extend his fingers. Master followed this up by lifting the opponent's foot off the ground. Master then said to him, "Don't be ashamed of your ability. Remember your many years of hard practice. Were it not for this, you would have been seriously injured." Master thus earned his deepest respect.

Late Master Wang Tsung-yüeh spread his art throughout eastern Chekiang and Honan, but Chekiang very early lost it. From Ch'en-chia-kou in Honan it was passed to Yang Lu-ch'an. After fifty years and several generations, the majority of T'ai-chi ch'üan practitioners are Yang stylists. It may be asked whether the Yang family maintained a complete monopoly in Yung-nien County? Although there are some other good practitioners, they were among the ten odd students of Yang Pan-hou. Therefore among practitioners of T'ai-chi ch'üan there are none who were not helped by Yang masters.

Some say that T'ai-chi ch'üan is of no practical use. Peking was formerly a magnet for all the martial heroes of China. Everyone called Master Yang Pan-hou, "Yang the Unbeatable." If you say you cannot throw someone with T'ai-chi, it is simply because your skill has not matured. Don't say that T'ai-chi is of no practical use. Don't be afraid of someone, even if they are as strong as a bull. If internal power cannot overcome strong opponents, why bother to study martial arts? When a thousand pounds lands on nothing it is useless.

Tung Ying-chieh's Secret Method

To use T'ai-chi you must know the time of day, the terrain, and human harmony.

The method relating to the time of day means that when squaring off with an opponent, do not face east in the morning, do not face south during midday, and do not face west in the evening. This is because one should avoid facing the sun.

The method relating to the terrain means that when squaring off with an opponent, first survey the lay of the land as to its spaciousness and elevation. It is most advantageous to occupy the lower ground.

The method of human harmony means that, although you are involved in a contest, you should be polite and not lose your dignity.

Today there are many styles of T'ai-chi ch'üan, and it is difficult for students to distinguish the good from the bad. Let me respectfully recommend a method. Regardless of the individual or the transmission, if they are capable of using both softness and hardness and of relaxing the sinews and invigorating the blood, they are correct. There is another method based on the civil and the martial. Observe their arms, and if the skin is very soft and the bones and flesh are very relaxed and heavy, this is correct. This is the civil method of ascertaining quality. When it comes to self-defense applications, we should look for the ability to use T'ai-chi methods and postures without confusion and to throw opponents while remaining perfectly at ease. This is the martial method of ascertaining quality. If the individual uses

144

force and flails wildly, he may be victorious, but it is strictly luck. This is not a true transmission and is really no method at all. Thus it is easy for students to recognize the true T'ai-chi ch'üan.

In T'ai-chi ch'üan, the ability to cultivate oneself physically and spiritually, but not to defend oneself, is civil accomplishment. The ability to defend oneself, but not to cultivate oneself, is martial accomplishment. The soft T'ai-chi method is the true T'ai-chi method. The ability to teach people the art of self-cultivation and self-defense, both cultivation and application, is complete civil and martial T'ai-chi.

The most important factors in determining an individual's strength or weakness are the *ch'i* and blood. Master Yang's style is open and relaxed and is best able to stretch the sinews and invigorate the blood. If those who are physically weak will practice Master Yang's style, they will see tremendous results.

In T'ai-chi there are "sinew-separating" and "bone-breaking" techniques; there are "pressure points," "*yin* hand and *yang* hand," "Five Elements hand," "bone penetrating" techniques, "the heart rending hammer," "tiger's eye elbow," "sticky mountain shoulder," "mandarin duck's leg," "sneaky seizing" techniques, and the ability to "beat a bull on the other side of the mountain." This does not mean literally beating a bull, but that without pain to the skin, internal damage can be inflicted.

T'ai-chi ch'üan is an internal system [*nei-chia ch'üan*]. It is popularly known as "Internal Boxing" [*nei-kung ch'üan*]. Among the martial arts, the internal system is the most dangerous. After students gain this skill, it is of the utmost importance to remain gentle and kind. Do not lightly use your full force to strike anyone or disgrace the legacy of former teachers.

T'ai-chi ch'üan enjoys great popularity in China now, and among martial artists all greatly value its practice. Nevertheless, every student has a different goal. If the object is simply physical exercise, then any teacher will do. However, if the goal is to learn self-defense, then a superior teacher is indispensable.

Practicing T'ai-chi ch'üan can strengthen the weak and rejuvenate the old. If you want timely results, avoid tobacco, alcohol and sex, and keep reasonable hours. Restrict all forms of harmful habits.

Transmission of the martial arts begins with two schools; Wutang and Shaolin. To this day they remain distinct. Even among those originating in the Shaolin Temple, there are a number of different systems, and the Wutang Mountains have also yielded their share. To say that they are all the same is impossible. If we speak only of T'ai-chi ch'üan, then most schools stem from Yang Lu-ch'an's transmission. At present it has divided into an Eastern School and a Western School, and each praises themselves to the skies. Beginnners will have great difficulty in determining relative merits. I may say that my art is the best, but in the end who can tell? Ideally one should be aware of the different postures. Some say they emphasize power, some say skill; but whatever the case, there can be only one set of principles. Without the true transmission, one cannot understand the reason for this.

———————

There are two methods of studying the martial arts. You can either study with friends who are roughly the same age, or seek out a teacher. With constancy both can lead to success.

———————

In the martial arts, the question of how much the teacher offers lies completely with the student, and not with the teacher. Let me explain briefly. Nowadays many people appreciate the value of T'ai-chi ch'üan and have a real desire to study, but they are skeptical about whether their teacher has the true transmission. Before they have even crossed the threshold they are already thirty percent afraid. Although the teacher would like to pass on his knowledge, what can he do?

Also, many students give up in mid-course, and then blame the teacher for not sharing his knowledge, without questioning their own study habits. This should be a warning to those who make such accusations against their teachers. We might compare this to the Three Kingdom's general, Liu Pei, who requested the service of K'ung Ming, but without asking if he was interested in coming out of seclusion or not. He asked once, twice, and three times, but K'ung Ming did not want to come out. How could Liu Pei secure talent in this way? This can serve as a lesson to students. I hope that colleagues will spread the art of T'ai-chi ch'üan and think about this.

———————

To learn something good you have to use your mind a little.

———————

147

If you gain something valuable from a book, don't claim that you invented it yourself, for this shows ingratitude to the author for his hard work.

———————

Master Yang was very open in transmitting his art. He taught everyone equally. Why then did some accomplish much and some little? It is because of differences in disposition, intelligence, and comprehension of the teaching. It is also because the principles in T'ai-chi are extremely profound and cannot be understood in one day. There are stages in progress to the top, and the teacher's method is to advance step by step. To abandon one's study before reaching the highest level, and then accuse the teacher of being an imposter is pure nonsense. Expecting to see nuggets of gold after a few days and little effort is also unrealistic. Keep on studying and there is no reason for the teacher not to give his knowledge freely.

———————

One day Master Yang was in the mood for fun and was demonstrating practical applications. He was pushing-hands with Wang Pao-huan, and using the Push technique, threw him for a distance of more than three yards. It was truly impressive. Master's self-defense was such that when pushing-hands with an opponent, it always seemed like they had no root in their feet and could not stand steadily. If you looked at Master, his countenance was perfectly composed and his hands and feet light and sensitive. But all he had to do was raise his hand and the opponent would fly with the speed of an arrow shot from a bow. Master Yang's technique was truly marvelous. None failed to respect him.

———————

T'ai-chi ch'üan is an internal system. If the postures are correct and the inner principles are understood, then this is T'ai-chi ch'üan. If the postures are not correct and the inner principles are not understood, even if the postures resemble T'ai-chi, there is no difference from the external systems.

The treasures of the ancient martial arts have surely not been transmitted intact. In the future, if those who tend to forget their teachers will hold on to the knowledge they have handed down, then we will surely receive the true transmission. This is indubitable.

Learning self-defense applications is indispensable in T'ai-chi ch'üan. Students who are primarily interested in exercise must also study applications. If they don't, it becomes very dull and the majority will quit. In fact, ignoring the applications is also an obstacle to making progress in strengthening the body.

The purpose of mastering self-defense applications is not to bully people, but to study the marvelous principles with friends. You attack and I neutralize; I attack and you respond. It flows on and on without end. Every kind of change can take place without exhausting the possibilities. If one realizes that there are infinite variations in T'ai-chi ch'üan, with dancing hands and stepping feet, then the interest increases daily. With practice over the years, this continuous and unforgettable joy greatly strengthens the body. To train the body it is important to study the applications, and even more so if one expects to face opponents. Therefore friends, when practicing T'ai-chi ch'üan, it is absolutely necessary to study the applications.

Chapter VIII

From Yang Ch'eng-fu's
Complete Principles and Applications of T'ai-chi ch'üan

Yang Ch'eng-fu,
T'ai-chi ch'üan t'i-yung ch'üan-shu
(Complete principles and
applications of T'ai-chi chüan),
Taipei: Chung-hua wu-shu
ch'u-pan-she, 1975
(first edition, 1934).

Yang Ch'eng-fu's Preface

In my youth I used to see my late grandfather, Yang Lu-ch'an, lead my paternal uncles and other students in daily practice of T'ai-chi ch'üan. They trained day and night without rest, both individually and in pairs. I was skeptical, however, believing self-defense against one man was not worth studying, and that in the future, I would study defense against ten thousand.

After I was a bit older, my late uncle, Yang Pan-hou, bid me study with him. As I could no longer conceal my doubts, I expressed them to him directly. My late father, Chien-hou, became angry and said, ''Well now, what kind of words are these? Your grandfather bequeathed this to our family. Do you propose to discard our family's heritage?'' My late grandfather, Lu-ch'an , calmed him saying, ''Children should not be coerced.'' He gave me a gentle pat and continued, ''Hold on for a minute and let me explain. The reason I practice and teach this art is not to challenge others but for self-defense, not to bully the world but to save the nation. The gentlemen of today know only of the poverty of the nation, but not of its weakness. Therefore our leaders anxiously formulate policies to alleviate poverty, but I have never heard of plans to rouse the weak or raise up the ailing. With a nation of sick people, who is equal to the task? We are poor because we are weak; truly weakness is the cause of poverty. If we examine the rise of nations, we find that they all begin by strengthening the people. The virility and vigor of the Europeans and Americans goes without saying, but the dwarf-like Japanese, while short in stature, are disciplined and determined. When the gaunt and emaciated members of our race face them, one need not resort to divination to predict the outcome. Thus the best method of saving the nation is to make saving the weak our highest priority. To ignore this is to be doomed to failure.

From my youth I have always considered helping the weak as my personal responsibility. I have seen popular martial arts performers whose spirit and physique are in no way inferior to the so-called muscle men of the West. With great enthusiasm I begged to learn their art, but they kept it secret and would not tell me. In this way I discovered that China's possessing the art of physical health and yet having become so weak is not without cause.

Still later I heard that at Ch'en-chia-kou in Honan there was a Ch'en family who were famous for their internal boxing and I made immediate haste to go there and study with Ch'en Ch'ang-hsing. Although I was not turned away at the door, after a long time I was still not allowed to share their secrets. I forbore and was patient for more than ten years. My teacher was moved by my sincerity and began, in the evenings when everyone else was resting, to reveal the secrets to me. After completing my studies I came to the capital and swore an oath to teach this art freely to all comers. Before long I saw that among my students, the thin filled out, the obese lost weight, and the sick became healthy. I was enormously gratified.

It seemed to me that what one individual could teach was limited and very like the foolish old man who tried to move the mountain. Also would not those of my elder's generation and those whose ambition was to play the bully look down upon this method of saving the nation and choose not to study it?'' At that moment I came suddenly to appreciate my grandfather's diligence in respect to this art and from then on dedicated myself to carrying on the family transmission. I eagerly submitted myself to training.

My grandfather had handed down these words: "T'ai-chi ch'üan began with Chang San-feng at the end of the Sung dynasty. He transmitted it to Wang Tsung-yüeh, Ch'en Chou-t'ung, Chang Sung-hsi and Chiang

Fa, who succeeded each other without interruption. My teacher, Ch'en Ch'ang-hsing, was the only disciple of Chiang-Fa. His art was based on the natural, and its form never departed from the Great Ultimate. It consisted of thirteen postures with infinite applications. The movement is in the body, but the influence reaches the spirit. Thus, without long practice, it is difficult to achieve the highest level. I have no shortage of students, but as for those who have been tempered to absolute perfection, I cannot even be certain of Pan-hou. However, if we speak only of the science of health, then one day's effort produces one day's benefit, and one year, one year's results. If you understand this, my child, then you possess the means to carry out my ambition.'' I respectfully observed his words and never dared forget them. From that point forward, I worked without ceasing for twenty years. My grandfather, uncle and father passed away one after the other.

At first I began to accept students in Peking but felt confined and limited in my results, so I traveled south to the Fukien-Chekiang region between the Yangtze and Huai Rivers. I later asked my student, Ch'en Wei-ming, to publish a book based on my oral instructions. Now ten years later, T'ai-chi ch'üan has spread north and south of the Yellow River and east and west of the Yangtze, even as far as Kwangtung Province. Altogether there are a great number of students. Ch'en's book explains only the sequence of solo practice, and looking back at the photographs of my postures ten years ago, they are inferior to today's. From this it can be seen that this art will continue to evolve indefinitely.

Today, at the request of my students, I have once again compiled the complete method of principles and applications, and added new photographs throughout. I have committed this to print in order to share it with the world. The techniques for two-edged sword, spear, two-pronged spear, broadsword, and so forth will be

presented in a second volume to follow. I do not dare to
seek fame through my art but humbly desire to further
my forebears' ambition to rouse the people and save the
world.

Written by Yang Chao-ch'ing (Ch'eng-fu)
of Kuang-p'ing in the spring of 1933.

Introduction

The guiding principle of this book lies in giving equal
importance to both principles and applications. The
number of people studying T'ai-chi ch'üan increases
daily. However, without understanding how to com-
bine principles and applications, there will be very little
benefit. Thus I have no thought for worldly gain, but
only the hope of finding brave and ambitious men who
are devoted to progress. Along with all my countrymen,
I wish to encourage them.

T'ai-chi ch'üan is based on the *I ching's* Great Ultimate
and eight trigrams. It develops out of the three concepts:
principle (*li*), *ch'i*, and form (*hsiang*). How can that which
Confucius referred to as, "embracing all the changes in
Heaven and earth without excess," be other than principle, *ch'i*, and form? Principle, *ch'i* and form are the origin
of T'ai-chi chüan. When these three are all developed,
then principle and application are complete. As for
form, it is modeled on the Great Ultimate and the eight
trigrams. *Ch'i* is nothing but *yin* and *yang*, hard and soft.
Principle controls that which is changeless in change
and is the root of transformation. Students should first
seek the proper form, in order to cultivate their *ch'i*.
After a time, they will naturally grasp the principles.

The essence of T'ai-chi ch'üan lies in the regulation of
movement and stillness. Thus in practicing, we must
observe the proper measure in the height of our stance,
the lightness or heaviness of our movement, the
extension and retraction of our advance or retreat, the

expansiveness or fineness of our breath, the direction of our gaze and the position of the waist, head, back and belly. It is an error to be suddenly high and suddenly low, suddenly fast and suddenly slow, suddenly light and suddenly heavy, to suddenly thrust and suddenly retract, to be suddenly large and suddenly fine, or to go suddenly left, right, up, down, facing upward or downward without evenness. Only when the height of our stance and the speed of our hands is guided by the proper measure can we be free of the necessity for fixed rules of height and speed.

Altogether there are thirteen important points for the practice of T'ai-chi ch'üan. These are: 1)Sink the shoulders and drop the elbows, 2)Depress the chest and raise the back, 3)Let the *ch'i* sink to the *tan-t'ien,* 4) The energy at the top of the head should be light and sensitive, 5) Relax the waist and hips, 6) Distinguish full and empty, 7) Coordinate the upper and lower body, 8) Use the mind and not force, 9) Harmonize the internal and external, 10) Connect the mind and *ch'i,* 11) Seek stillness in movement, 12) Unify movement and stillness, 13) Each posture should be even and uniform. These are the thirteen points. We must pay attention to every movement. Every posture must be precise. Not one of these thirteen concepts can be overlooked. I hope that students will maintain a careful and critical attitude.

The self-defense applications in this book are intended for those who are already thoroughly trained in T'ai-chi ch'üan and would like to make further progress. Thus they need not be restricted as to which direction to face and can experiment with the four sides and four corners of the square. Those who are not familiar with the form should not advance to the applications, for without a solid foundation there will be few results. I hope that beginners will carefully study the postures shown in the illustrations. When one has become adept at the form, it will not be difficult to master the applications.

There is only one school of T'ai-chi ch'üan; there are not two methods. Don't be deluded by your own cleverness and foolishly make additions or deletions. If modifications were necessary in the methods laid down by worthy men of the past, then these would have been implemented during the many centuries from the Yüan and Ming dynasties down to the present. Did these modifications need to wait for our own generation? I hope that future students will not be led astray by externals, but seek always the inner truth. One must be patient if one desires to advance to the highest excellence. The most important thing in studying the postures is not the external appearance, but to grasp the idea. The greatest danger is in introducing one's personal innovations and passing on errors as true transmissions. The true transmission of principles and applications is easily lost, even to the point of obscuring the original intention of former masters. Thus we offer this book, which is based on the old texts with revisions, as a correct standard.

T'ai-chi ch'üan was not created merely to brawl with ruffians. Rather, the Immortal, Chang San-feng, invented this soft martial art as an aid to maintaining good health. Those who are interested in health and self-discipline, eliminating illness and lengthening years, whether men of letters, in poor health, as well as old people, the young and women, all may study. Those who practice faithfully will see real results in three years. If one should ask about its usefulness, the answer is that it allows us to use no strength and yet not be intimidated by strength. If someone possessed of great strength should attack us, then our supreme softness is sufficient to defeat them. We succeed by following the opponent's force. We might say that the key to health and self-discipline lies in following and preserving weakness. Even the ferocious strength of such ancient warriors as Meng Pen and Hsia Yü is of no interest to practitioners of

T'ai-chi ch'üan.

When beginning to study the T'ai-chi form, one must absolutely avoid haste. Every day thoroughly practice one or two postures and it will be easy to appreciate their inner essence. Those who practice too much at one time can only scratch the surface. After finishing one's practice, do not immediately sit down, but walk about a bit in order to readjust the *ch'i* and blood.

After practicing in the heat of summer, do not wash the hands with cold water or one will be "afflicted by fire." After practicing in the cold of winter, quickly put on warm clothing in order to avoid catching cold. One's skill will increase during the winter and summer. This is why it is said, "Train during the three periods after the summer solstice and the three periods after the winter solstice." At these times the sun's influence is more powerful than during the spring and autumn. It is absolutely essential not to neglect practice just after rising and just before retiring. In this way one's skill will easily show progress.